Seeing through a Glass Darkly

A Guide to Healing from Childhood Trauma

By Julie Anne Wankier
with Tere Weir

Cover art by De Lanie Beus Heath
Scriptures quoted are from the King James Version Bible

ISBN 0-9721283-0-1
Copyright © 2002
Published in the U.S.A.

*For now we see through a glass, darkly; but
then face to face: now I know in part; but
then shall I know even as also I am known.*

1 Corinthians 13:12

DEDICATION

This book is dedicated to my father who believes it is the secret, not the truth that hurts us. With clean hands my father stands with my mother in support of all who will come unto Christ and be healed.

A NOTE TO THE READER

Although this book is written with specific examples about sexual abuse, the principles of how to heal and receive wholeness apply to anyone whose pain stems from childhood. If you are trying to heal or forgive or repent, read further. Parts of this book may be applicable to your situation.

I have liberally used the scriptures throughout the book. I have tried to write truth as I know it by likening the scriptures to myself. This is how I learned and discovered healing. These are my impressions of truth

You will notice as you read the book that victims are designated as female and perpetrators as designated as male. I realize that victims and perpetrators can be male or female. I have simply designated gender to avoid confusion in reading.

FOREWORD

A couple of years ago, I listened as a gentleman spoke of the sacrifice of our great ancestors. My mind opened to the sacrifice and pain many experienced as they left their homeland for safety, freedom of worship, or happiness. I saw the courage and strength it took.

Symbolically, I saw people crossing a wilderness of healing from abuse. They were tired. The road was long and hard to travel. The way was difficult to follow. I felt impressed that God would need people to help to lift them, strengthen them, and move them on their way.

Then I saw the advancements of time. I saw trails much easier to travel, then railroads and train travel. Finally I saw planes which made the journey quicker. I hope following the path of someone who has healed from abuse will make your path to healing an easier one to follow. I pray with all my heart to add to the beautiful work of others who have paved the beginning trails of healing. I see the promise of smoother paths and more rapid travel to heal the wounded hearts of those who innocently suffer.

This book is not a substitute for other self-help books. Reading self-help books helped me to heal and by applying principles in those books I feel the Lord has helped me to learn more.

God gives light and truth to His children to help them with physical difficulties. He also assists with mental and emotional problems–problems that hold them back spiritually from reaching their promised land. How grateful I am to God for giving light and truth to help us in our life.

I hope this book will lead you to see prayer and scripture study in a new light, with new eyes. I hope that you will long to use the ways of the Lord to heal and that instead of feeling ostracized by God, you will feel embraced by Him.

God bless you as you read this book. I hope the Holy Spirit will move you to know God's will for you, His love for you, and the Savior's healing that awaits you.

TABLE OF CONTENTS

CHAPTER ONE

SEEING BROKEN GLASS ALL AROUND ME

*"By sorrow of the heart the spirit is broken"
(Proverbs 15:13).*

Do you ever wonder why life seems difficult? Do your days hold more than you can handle? Do you make decisions based on fear of what others will think? Do you please others rather than act on how you feel toward yourself? Do you have trouble sleeping or do you turn to sleep as an escape? Does the pain inside seem to have been there ever since your life began?

If you feel some of these feelings, you may have collided with your past which is breaking your ability to move happily in your today. If you are unable to connect with the happiness for which you long, you may need to look at the pain that is getting in your way. When you face your pain, your reality may shatter into pieces. Because of childhood trauma, you may realize you have survived a reality that has held you back or barely moving forward from day to day.

When you allow yourself to learn about how your present is being affected by the past, you can begin to open up a new world of viewing yourself, God, and the world around you. This chapter will teach you about some of the effects of the "broken glass" inside yourself. Take courage, dealing with the "broken glass" inside will help you break the cycle of barely functioning. Then you can move toward lasting wholeness and healing.

THE SPECTRUM OF CHILDHOOD TRAUMA

What kinds of experiences cause childhood trauma? What can be done to help a child or adult heal from childhood trauma?

Childhood trauma is experiencing pain severe enough that it not only affects your childhood and your development as a child, the pain may also affect your adulthood. The various types of trauma cover a wide spectrum of ages and experience.

Childhood trauma may occur any time from birth to somewhere between 19-21 years of age. Because each age is essential to the development and foundation of who you are, when you experience trauma during your childhood, your development can be affected in adverse ways. It is important to note that some adults continue to experience trauma after they are grown, and because it connects to their childhood trauma it can still be considered childhood trauma.

What causes childhood trauma? Childhood trauma is caused in many ways. Natural disasters are one example. A child experiences trauma by being victim to natural catastrophes such as earthquakes, floods, or famine. This trauma of experiencing or seeing people fearful, hurt, or dying requires a level of understanding too high for a child to work through. Such intense experiences require internalizing truth using adult or abstract thinking.

Trauma from perpetrators. Children who have evil acts perpetrated on them also experience childhood trauma. These acts include sexual, physical, emotional, mental, and spiritual abuse. Children require high-level teaching to heal from this type of abuse.

Other evil practices are called Satanic Ritual Abuse. In

this type of abuse authority figures attempt to gain power in "religious" settings, drug cults, and secret clubs. These types of practices cause extreme trauma in children. Healing must come through the love and guidance of an adult who can nurture, teach truth, and patiently listen to the person's traumatic experience in order to help in healing.

Other traumatic experiences. Children who are neglected may suffer from childhood trauma. Physical difficulties may also cause trauma: hospitalizations, surgeries, accidents, extended and severe illnesses require nurturing and teaching to help the child feel safe in life. Children who live in a country that is in war or unrest may experience severe trauma-- especially if they witness violence and death firsthand.

How to use this book. This book, though focused on the evil acts of abuse that cause childhood trauma, can be best used if the ideas are applied to all different types of trauma, forces of nature, health issues, war, as well as those issues specific to abuse. If you have pain that links to childhood experience, learn and apply the principles of this book and you will give yourself the gift of discovering a newness of life. You will find the joy and peace that are locked inside behind the pain and confusion of the inner self.

Conclusion:
1. Childhood trauma is pain that impacts your childhood, your development, and possibly your adulthood.
2. Trauma can be caused in many different ways. Disasters, abuse, war, and health problems are a few examples.

THE BROKEN INNER SELF

Sometimes I think I hear voices. Am I crazy?
Who is the inner child I need to nurture?

Throughout this book you will read the term "inner child." It is important to understand exactly what the term means. Inner children are created because of trauma. An inner child can be found in your subconscious feelings. Traumatic childhood experiences, emotions, and thinking are held frozen in time. These experiences and ways of thinking color the way you look at the world, the way you respond to others, and how you react to daily situations.

You may not even realize the inner child is there and at times you may be surprised at how you act. There may be times when you react far more emotionally than warranted by the circumstances and you may wonder why.

This all has to do with past experiences and your memories of those experiences. You may be blessed to have peaceful childhood memories of good nurturing, family work ethic, family traditions, gospel learning and love. Other memories, however, may be traumatic and painful experiences which have broken your heart like shattered glass creating an inner child or inner children.

Trauma during childhood causes a lack of progression during development. Look at the following chart. See how at different ages traumatic experience breaks the healthy progression of the developmental stage of the child.

Trauma during Development Causes Lack of Progression
Erikson's Social Interaction

0–1 year
Trust vs. Mistrust
Sees world as safe if people
are helpful and dependable. If
care is inconsistent, this creates
an attitude of fear and suspicion.*

2–3 years
Autonomy vs. Doubt
Develops a sense of being able to control
muscles, impulses, oneself and one's environment. If
caretaker is harsh and unthinking, the child develops an excessive
sense of shame with respect to other people and an excessive sense
of doubt about one's own abilities to control one's world and oneself.

4–5 years
Initiative vs. Guilt
Stage where social actions are initiated. This stage is left when the
child given much freedom and opportunity to initiative activities. When
made to feel an activity is bad, then guilt will override.

6–11 years
Industry vs. Inferiority
Child becomes capable of deductive reasoning. The child succeeds when
given freedom to learn how things are made, how they work, and what they
do. If the child experiences constant failures in academic efforts, it reinforces
a sense of inferiority. The child no longer depends solely on the care giving
efforts of the parents, but on the actions of other adults as well.

12–18 years
Identity vs. Role Confusion
Child's task is to bring together all things learned about being a son or daughter,
student, friend, etc. and integrate these different images into a whole that makes
sense and that shows continuity with the past while preparing for the future.
The influence of parents is indirect. When the child cannot attain a sense of
personal identity either because of an unfortunate childhood or difficult social
circumstances, role confusion results.

*Note: This dimension is not resolved once and for all during the first year. The
conflicts arise again at each successive stage. The problems of a past stage must be
conquered in the successive stages. Trauma in a later stage can undo the progress
of the previous stages, but successful experiences at a later stage can heal past
problems. Based on Erik Erikson's Eight Ages of Man.

Responding to childhood memories. Almost everyone has experienced something when they were young that surfaces in the way they react to events or stimuli as an adult. Instead of acting on a conscious level, they react on a subconscious emotional level. When you react emotionally, you could be responding to a childhood memory. Reacting because of feelings instead of responding with rational thinking shows a brokenness within. You are influenced by inner conflict as you choose how you deal with life.

Because of these painful memories, you respond to non-threatening situations as though you are threatened. When your inner child is wounded, your pain radiates out to others-- your children, neighbors, church and family members, and God. You may treat others the way you were treated. The inner child is calling for help, not knowing how to be heard, understood, or helped.

Your inconsistent behavior is an expression of the intense feelings caused from previous pain and confusion. Suppose in fifth grade a boy tells the class you are stupid. You feel humiliated. Years later, if your competence is questioned, you may respond the way you did to the fifth grade boy. This bad experience causes an inner child reaction at a later time. Your inner self believed what the boy said and internalized it. When you have a similar experience as an adult, your inner child hears, "You are stupid," and reacts to the emotional pain.

When you experience abuse as a child, you experience trauma which affects your inner child. Imagine again you are in fifth grade. A perpetrator is controlling you. As a perpetrator approaches to abuse you, you respond by freezing (the most common response). You feel paralyzed and unable to leave or protect yourself.

Your perpetrator's actions lie saying, "You have no worth. I can do anything I want to you and you can't stop me.

6

You are less important than I am. In fact, you are to blame because you are not leaving. You want what I am demanding."

As an adult, when someone tries to control you, your inner child may scream, "If this person gets what he wants, he's controlling me and I am worthless and to blame." The anxious feelings will be so loud that you will respond by controlling so you can find calmness within. These feelings, experiences, and ways of thinking need to be worked through so you can act for yourself instead of reacting based on emotion. (See *Control Issues, p. 23.*)

Does trauma from your childhood affect your daily life? Look at whether you act or react to life situations. Do you make decisions based on fears, feelings of low self-worth or a belief that does not correspond with faith and gospel truth? Do you do things because you can't feel calm about other decisions that logically appear to be good?

My broken inner self affected my dating years. I married at age 27, so I saw a pattern of acting versus reacting as I dealt with the issue of sexual boundaries. My religious beliefs taught me to be morally clean. This meant no sexual relations or anything like it. When asked on a date I would decide to have an uplifting, wholesome evening. I worked to plan activities conducive to that.

Then my date would hold my hand or put his arm around me. The anxiety would start. I would feel I was expected to do what he wanted and I had no ability to follow my great plans. I felt I was alone waging a war inside of myself.

One part of me would say, "You can't kiss him or you are in trouble." Another part of me would believe I had no control. A part of me would believe I could read the young man's mind and know he wanted to kiss me. I felt I must kiss him, feeling paralyzed to do anything else.

The pain inside of me escalated as I remembered my lofty goals, how I hoped to have an uplifting evening. I would feel I had ruined the evening. I would feel unsafe and trapped, like I was being attacked. I would even feel like I was in trouble with God because I should have known the night would lead to some type of physical relationship, though for me this meant only a kiss or a hug.

I would promise myself to do what I needed to do the next time, but I knew I was in trouble. I would tell myself I could never get myself in this situation again or I could never be a good person. I felt bad to the core.

After a date I would look at myself in the mirror and see a blank stare, an empty shell. I was trapped within and trapped without. I would create stories for myself of how I conquered my weakness and accomplished good so as to avoid facing my helpless self.

Time and time again I prayed to God for help and would feel I should not go out with the same young man any more. These impressions kept me from ever having a sexual relationship during my single years, but I continued to be without boundaries until I healed during therapy which helped me work through confused feelings and distorted beliefs.

My inner child was the source of feelings that did not match up with my desires. I didn't seem to have full freedom to act on what I knew I wanted when life experience collided with inner feelings. The broken children inside of me held the feelings that motivated what I did. Those feelings came from a deeply embedded belief of whom I was based on example and experience from others during the foundation of my life. These feelings formed who I believed I was.

Discovering the inner child. Many people do not realize they have an inner brokenness. Often people only learn to recognize the inner child, because they are experiencing pain in the form of confusion, depression, anxiety, bad dreams, and numbness. When these emotions dominate their life, they attempt to discover what is wrong. Then they open the door to discovering feelings stuck within.

> *Mar. 21, 1988. I've felt very trapped inside myself like the real Julie Anne is trapped in a shell of what she thinks she ought to be and is trying to come out. I have a great capacity to love somewhere inside of me, but fears and a lack of trust smother it. I have a hard time giving when I'm so "inside myself."*

You might discover an inner child by closing your eyes to allow yourself to visualize what is happening inside. As you relax you will see, not create, what is happening. At first it will seem like your imagination. The goal is to find what is inside and bring it from the dark to the Savior. This will not always work because not every problem stems from childhood, but it is a good place to start.

Once you have discovered your inner child, you can start to teach her and help her heal. In a spiritual perspective, the inner child wonders who she is. The inner child that has been hurt doesn't feel a wonderful feeling associated with being a follower of Christ. You can teach your inner child about faith in God. You can be the facilitator in helping your inner child heal. (See *Parenting the Inner Child*, p. 123.)

As you learn to listen to your inner child, you will discover pain and trauma trapped inside you. You can start to heal the inner child and finally find peace for yourself.

Conclusion:

1. The inner child is the feelings, trauma, and

experiences frozen in time within yourself.

    2. The voices you hear inside yourself are your inner child responding to your present situation from her perspective.

    3. The inner child will respond to situations at the developmental level she was at when the trauma occurred.

MORAL LIMBO

    How can I learn to do things for the right reasons? What are the "right reasons" for living a moral life?

What does it mean to live a moral life? This means being honest and having integrity. It means treating others and ourselves with love and respect. It means making good choices for the right reasons.

Kohlberg's teachings on Moral Education. Inspired by Piaget, Kohlberg studied moral development and discovered some amazing truths about how we progress in choosing the right. He teaches there is a hierarchy in making choices and we learn to make choices on different levels as we grow and progress.

    For instance, a small child may choose to do a job her mother asks her to because she wants to earn a treat or to avoid being sent to her room. If the treat isn't offered or the punishment threatened, the child may not choose to do the job.

    A more mature child acts on a higher level of thinking. She might think, *If I do this job, my mother will do something for me.* She sees benefits come from her choice. On the highest level, a child will do a service simply because she loves her mother and wants to show her love. The following chart shows this hierarchy of thinking.

10

Christ-Centered Healing
Opens up Eternal Progression

Kohlberg
Moral Education Stages

6. The Universal Ethical Principle Orientation. "Do unto others as you would have others do unto you." (Charity)
Note: Number 6 was dropped from the measure because the testers did not find any examples.

5. Social Contract, Human Rights, and Welfare Orientation. Defines right action in terms of general individual rights. Example: U.S. Constitution.

4. Societal Maintenance Orientation. Follow fixed rules, respect authority.

3. Interpersonal Sharing Orientation. Earn approval by being nice.

2. Instrumental Relativist Orientation. "You scratch my back and I'll scratch yours."

1. Punishment vs. Obedience. Think about avoiding punishment or earning rewards.

These stages are often set during the first half of life. However, during a time of trial and healing, conflict in the mind of the individual forces the child to use higher-stage reasoning to solve problems. When exposed to one stage higher than the child's own level, growth will be enhanced. Based on Kohlberg's Moral Education for Young Children.

Making choices for the right reasons. When you make moral choices, you don't simply refrain from choosing evil. You make good choices for good reasons. When you make bad choices--or even good choices for lower level reasons than you are capable--you thwart your progress. When you choose the right for base reasons, your soul does not gain the strength it needs to withstand evil.

One of the reasons you may struggle with this is because your inner child may be stuck at a young developmental stage. You make choices influenced by your inner child. This is why it is so important to parent your inner child and help her grow developmentally. (See *Parenting the Inner Child, p. 123*.)

If you are making choices based on one of the lower moral stages, you may obey God's commandments to avoid punishment, to receive blessings, or to be praised. When you are obedient for these reasons, you may not be able to maintain the course you would like to follow because you lack strength to face the great opposition in the world today. You must make good choices for higher reasons.

It is not enough to obey God or follow church leaders because you respect their authority. If you live God's ways only to be obedient, you may find that opposition or affliction causes you to waver. For example, you are obedient and so you expect God to bless you. When a trial comes into your life, you become mad at God and feel He isn't being fair to you.

The highest option: making good choices out of love. Charity is the best reason for doing good. When you live by charity, you are obedient to God's principles because you love God. In fact, God instructed, "If ye love me, keep my commandments" (John 14:15). You can be obedient to God because you love Him; and one way of showing you love Him is by your obedience.

12

It is imperative that you follow God with an internalized belief system that is riveted on the Savior's greatest attribute, love. You choose to follow God because you love Him with all your heart and long to be like Him. To heal will mean facing the hardest challenges of opposition and heartache you may ever face. You will be stretched to love in a way beyond your present capacity.

The greatest trial of not healing from abuse is you stay stuck in the lower stages of living truth. You follow truth to avoid punishment, to receive from others, to avoid looking bad, to avoid breaking rules and being disrespectful to those in authority. Although you benefit from avoiding negative in your life when you are motivated this way, when you live higher moral stages, you gain the freedom of living truth for the most rewarding reasons of all–to be like Christ and gain eternal life. Through healing you can reach higher moral levels and ultimately live near God because of your love for good.

Conclusion:
1. When you make good choices for the wrong reasons, your progress is thwarted.
2. The best choices are based on charity.

DISTORTED THINKING
Why do I seem to see life differently than other people?

How can I tell if I am looking at life the way it really is?

Distorted thinking is a natural consequence of abuse. You may have distorted thinking about how to relate to others and how to relate to God. Some distorted thinking helped you survive when you were a child, but now Satan uses distorted thinking as a wedge in your life to keep you at a distance from God and others. Distorted thinking leaves you weak, vulnerable, and unable to progress.

Examples of distorted thinking. You will find a heading listed after each example. Each example of distorted thinking is examined in greater detail in that section.

- You are responsible for the actions of others. (See *Guilt, p. 220*.)
- You can't trust God. (See *Feeling Abandoned by God, p. 204*.)
- You can't trust other people. (See *No One Will Save Me; Where Is My Savior? p. 205*.)
- You feel you are vulnerable and in constant danger even though everything around you appears fine. (See *Adult and Inner Child Conflict. p. 119*.)
- You feel doomed to do evil repeatedly. (See *Second Sins, p. 171*.)
- You can't be consistently happy. (See *Depression, p. 31*.)
- You are endlessly working, but feel unworthy for good or to be good. (See *Perfectionism, p. 27*.)
- You are a victim to other people. (See *The Family Secret, p. 158*.)
- You feel basically bad. (See *Shame, p. 224*.)
- You have to control or be controlled. (See *Control Issues, p. 23*.)

Ridding yourself of distorted thinking. How did distorted thinking help you survive as a child? Survival thinking helped the child cope and function. For instance, if you thought you were responsible for your perpetrator's actions, you had hope you could change your circumstances. This helped you feel life might change for the better and so helped you to survive the abuse. (See *Guilt, p. 220*.)

Now you need truth to help you heal from what happened. You need to discover distorted thinking and replace those distorted ideas with truth. Think of distorted thinking as a mistyped recipe you must adjust to cook a successful product. You must look at it logically to decide if flour, sugar, cinnamon, and mustard can successfully be used together to make cookies.

As you examine the recipe ask yourself, "What do I understand from my knowledge of food combinations to guess how this will taste? Are some of the ingredients correct? Which ones will ruin the recipe and what should replace those ingredients?" Decide what to keep and what to discard.

When you examine your thinking patterns, question yourself the same way. Examine your ideas and beliefs and decide whether they will create true thinking in your mind or whether they should be discarded. You may reorganize your beliefs and combine them in a new way. Damaging beliefs that have been stuffed in your mind must be discarded completely in order for the recipe of healing to be complete. This may cause discomfort for a time, but eventually you will be able to live by new truths.

As you act on what you know and not on how you feel, your inner self will begin to gain a testimony of your knowledge. This will come from seeing the positive outcomes which will align with truths you are applying.

Don't be discouraged if you feel you are in an upheaval while you are examining your beliefs. You are! You may feel you are regressing rather than progressing for awhile. This can happen when you evaluate your values and beliefs. But it is comforting to know that when you replace distortions with truth, you are replacing chaos and darkness with order and peace.

Distorted thinking about God. I looked at God two

different ways in my life--one way before healing and another way after healing. Before I healed, I had the distorted view that God expected me to be perfect in everything I said and did. I believed if I could become perfect, I would find peace. I thought I was living righteously only if I was doing everything perfectly. I felt God had no mercy nor reward for me unless I appeared perfect to others and to Him. (See *Perfectionism, p. 27.*)

I had to be doing, doing, doing. I hoped to "do-come" like God. Doing can sabotage healing. Just because you become an intense "[doer] of the word" (James 1:22) does not mean you internalize the true meaning of the word. Thus you may not receive promised blessings of peace for what you do.

September 14, 1993. I had a dream I was a man. I was standing in a grove of trees trying to combat Satan. I was doing all kinds of things to combat him. I would jump high in the air and spin to get away from him. Nothing worked. Each great attempt was defeated and Satan was in my face as strong as ever. I was tiring from working so hard, but I kept <u>doing</u> more and more.

Finally something stopped me. Satan was stronger then ever--defeating me--and something stopped me. The Spirit whispered to my soul, "You can't <u>do</u> anything--you must stand firm. This is an internal battle. Do you have internally what it takes to conquer Satan? Are you strong enough within to defeat him?" Then I woke up.

This dream put fear into my heart. I woke at 3:00 a.m. feeling far from peaceful. I scooted over by Brian, my husband, and told him my dream. I realize that this dream was symbolic of my life. I am busily <u>doing</u> many good things, but I am not internally spending balanced time praying, pondering, and studying the word of God.

This last couple of weeks I've done better.

Spiritually, I've fed myself better. I am far from my goal, but I know that line upon line I can become strong enough to stand firm in combat with Satan.

Jan. 9, 1994. Now I've learned even my relationship with God is distorted. This makes me feel paralyzed in my relationship with Him. Will He listen to me if I try to talk to him? How far away is He? Is He angry with me? Doesn't He see me trying?

Father, if you're there, please forgive me. I still don't feel at peace with Thee, so I feel I must have done something wrong. I often wonder what is real and I feel such anxiety about making choices about what I should do or not do. I wonder if I see things clearly.

I have so very far to go, so very much to learn. I feel so tired. Brian said I've said this since he met me–I've felt it for that long, I'm sure. I need to see things from a new perspective.

You are to "be-come" like God, not "do-come" like God. You should be motivated by what God is, not just what He does. When you are motivated by the knowledge of who you are and who God is, then you do what God needs to build His kingdom. You do good things to accomplish God's work and glory which is to return to God and help others get there too.

You do not need to prove your worth to God. In other words, don't overdose on doing while you learn to be the incredible being that God will teach you that you are in the silent moments of pondering and reflection.

God loves unconditionally. Upon healing I found my Father in Heavenly is a God of love. I discovered we are

17

worthy of our Savior's love simply because we are His children. We don't <u>do</u> anything to gain His love. He loves us, even when we make mistakes. His love is unconditional. (See *Feeling God Does Not Love Me, p. 209.*)

God accepts and loves me--imperfections and all. God allowed me weaknesses and difficult experiences to humble me so I would come to him. God cares about the direction I am heading. He wants me to progress toward Him. If I am moving toward Him, I am becoming more perfect. Perfection is a goal to be achieved step by step into eternity.

I learned that my interpretation of perfection was not God's interpretation. God doesn't worry about how things appear to others, He sees them as they really are. I learned that people do not get to judge our perfection, God does that.

Distorted thinking about repentance. Many victims have another distorted view of God. When they hear a call to repentance, they see God's condemnation upon them. They feel unworthy and believe God sees them as unworthy. They are feeling what the perpetrator should be feeling. The perpetrator is to experience the consequence of needing to repent.

A victim may feel God's words of condemnation and punishment, meant for the perpetrator, are meant for her. The victim needs to heal because of being bruised, broken, and torn--spiritually, mentally and emotionally. Thus, the victim sees God from a broken state and is unable to see His ways clearly. Those who need the healing word of God feel they receive chastisement.

I am sure church clergy worry about this very thing when they teach their people about repentance. These leaders are grieved they must be so bold speaking about wickedness and abominations, in the presence of the pure in heart and the broken hearted.

The broken hearted feel daggers piercing their souls and wounding their minds as they study the scriptures and read bold commands of the prophets written to the wicked. Their wounds are enlarged as they apply these strict words to their inner child selves. They misinterpret how God's word applies to them. (See *How Does God Ask Your Adult Self to View Your Inner Child? p. 217.*)

However, if prophets had preached the pleasing word of God instead of calling the wicked to repentance, the wicked may have believed they were being justified and could get away with sin. Just as prophets of old were required to cry repentance, church clergy today often do the same.

Abuse victims must realize they are not being called to repent for their perpetrator's sins. Adults repent as they make choices. When we have no choice or are children, we are innocent. (See *Ironic Similarities between Repenting and Healing,.* p. 286.)

While abuse victims suffer from many types of distorted thinking, these distorted views can be cleared up through healing. As the child self heals, the abuse victim will be able to look at relationships with God and others in a new light.

Conclusion:

1. Distorted thinking may help a child survive abuse, but adults need to get rid of distorted thinking so they can heal.

2. Getting rid of distorted thinking will not be an easy process. You may feel you are going backward for a time.

3. Many of your views will change as you get rid of distorted thinking.

FEELING MISUNDERSTOOD

Why do so many church teachings fill me with pain?

Why do answers to questions affect my feelings rather than my logic?

Because abusive relationships are dysfunctional relationships, you may struggle to know how you should feel about certain relationships in your life. For you, a mother/daughter relationship has a different meaning than for someone in a non-abusive situation. You may have difficulty with father/daughter, brother/sister relationships as well.

Because your inner child is in pain, you will process information differently than you would if you were not in pain. When you ask a question, you may <u>hear</u> one answer but <u>feel</u> another. You interpret answers in ways they were never intended to be felt.

Destructive relationships color other relationships. Many victims were abused by an older brother. Ideally older brothers represent a protector, a friend, an example to a younger sibling. When abuse occurs, the event damages not only the brother/sister relationship, but any relationship with the same symbolic characteristics.

How is the abuse victim going to view her relationship with the elder brother that atoned for her sins? She may feel abandoned by Him and have a difficult time trusting and embracing Jesus, her elder brother. It may be difficult to believe that He loves her and is her Exemplar and Redeemer. The inner child takes the pain from the abusive relationship and applies it to other similar relationships.

You can imagine the consequences if a father or grandfather is abusive. The victim is going to struggle with a relationship with Father in Heaven. If a neighbor was abusive, it is going to be painful to hear counsel to "love thy neighbor." (See *Feeling Abandoned by God, p. 204 .*)

Church hymns, sermons, lessons, and even everyday discussions can leave a victim feeling baffled and confused, empty and alone as she tries to figure out how to fit truth into her everyday life.

Processing information through the inner child's pain. When the truths a victim has learned in her mind do not match with the feelings in her heart, she tries to search for answers. She may dare ask a teacher or a friend a question like, "Why is God an angry God?" or "Why does God want us to fear Him?" She wonders "Why doesn't God answer my prayers?" or "Why does God help repentant people, but He doesn't help those that are hurt?"

The answers to these questions and many others will come the way the listener views it--coming to a sinful, unworthy adult. The answers will likely instill great pain and confusion to the sinless inner child.

Dec. 5, 1993. My perspective of myself being an abuse victim is holding me back from trusting others, opening up to friendships, and feeling understood. I feel protective of my abused self and can't seem to bridge the gap between this and being open to others.

Once I dared to share with a teacher a deep feeling from my inner self that for the first time I realized God wanted us to follow Him because we loved Him, not because we feared the consequences of disobedience. The teacher's answer was harsh to the ears of my inner child. He said God would not excuse the least amount of disobedience.

My inner self was already guilt ridden with consequences from my childhood pain. I (my inner child) needed to have hope that I was loved unconditionally. I felt like consequences were punishment to my inner self for being innately evil. I felt I could never be good enough to receive love.

My inner children were filled with increased pain. They felt they were evil and had hoped God could love them rather than want to see them continue to suffer. My inner children were stuck in pain. I heard a different answer than the one intended.

Confusion comes from the inner child stuck and being unable to see beyond immediate pain. This limitation can cause an endless feeling of being misunderstood. Your inner child needs you, your adult self, to re-parent her, to teach truth to help free her. Others cannot and do not know what is happening inside you. You must learn to clarify what others say and nurture your inner self.

When you consciously face pain your soul hasn't yet stretched to comprehend, you have two choices. You can either turn to the world and change truth to fit your circumstances or you can hold to the word of God and work to understand truth to the point where you can internalize your learning and change your feelings. You must progress to the point that your learning overrides your confusion and you gain understanding.

Conclusion:

1. When you interpret relationships around you based on former dysfunctional relationships in your life confusion results.

2. You might misunderstand the meaning of what people tell and teach you because you filter what they say

through a lens of distorted thinking.

    3. As you parent and heal your inner child, the feelings of being misunderstood will diminish.

CONTROL ISSUES

    Why do I feel I always lose?
    Why must I be in control to feel safe?

    In the midst of abuse there is no other feeling more helpless than to be controlled by someone. The victim feels she has no rights or power to say or do what she needs and wants. She feels degraded, thinking that she exists merely to fulfill an evil purpose.

    The reality is victims don't have control in an abusive relationship. They are in the relationship to gratify the abuser's pride or vain ambition. The abuser seeks to exercise control or dominion over his victim. The Spirit of the Lord is grieved by these acts.

    Control or be controlled. The controlled victim is blessed to survive, but learns that life offers two scenarios-- either control or be controlled. A victim may feel so much anxiety about the terror of being controlled that anytime she feels like someone might take away her agency, her instant impulse is to gain freedom or power by controlling the situation herself. She feels a need to control every aspect of her life.

    Feb. 10, 1991. No matter what Brian does, I'm unhappy. If he comes, I want to ignore him. If he leaves, I cry. I want to control his life and I want his life to revolve around mine. I've been so insecure about how I feel about myself and him. Something sets me off and I get angry, my jaw sets, my heart is full of anger and I withdraw love and affection from him.

On the other hand, some survivors feel there is no hope of ever rising above being controlled. They continue to allow others to control their life and have no aspirations to live as they desire. They have no feeling of self worth, no ability to rise above the acts of others. They continue to feel and act like a victim.

April, 13, 1988. Last Friday and Saturday I was with Nick, my fiance, and it was wonderful. I felt such a romantic love for him. I didn't want it to end but it did and now I feel I don't want to be with him.

The reason why? I wish I could say exactly. I think it has to do with being forced into small physical things I don't want to do. Nick puts my body where he wants it. If he wants me to put my head on his shoulder, he puts it there. If he wants me to lie down, he lays me down. I just can't deal with it.

Finding a balance. Because power should be controlled by using principles of righteousness, you must learn to act righteously by finding a balance between being controlled and being controlling. You must seek to give and receive. You can learn to allow others to act and express their thoughts without fearing that you will lose control if they gain it for a time. You do not need to feel you are "conquered" if you are not in charge.

How do you find that balance? You must learn you have a right to share opinions, beliefs, inspiration, and desires without feeling bad or self centered. You must also learn that to give and receive is a gift of being on earth. This means that others have a right to share their feelings and beliefs and doing this should not be a threat to you. As you learn this truth you can learn to give and receive love realizing that honest sharing will not hurt others.

You can learn to give through God's example.
God knows how to give good gifts to his children (see Matt. 7:11). "For God so loved the world, that he gave his only begotten Son, that whosoever believeth in him should not perish, but have everlasting life" (John 3:16).

When God sent His Son to earth as a sacrifice for our sins He gave the greatest gift ever given. There is no greater gift ever to be given, no greater gift to receive. There is a two-part plan to this gift. We believe in God and follow Him, then we receive everlasting life. (See *Trust, p. 240; Submission, p. 244.*)

God does not want to control you, but He does hope you will use agency in obedience. Love should be the foundation of this obedience. You do what is right when acting and being acted upon because you love and are loved. This way you are part of win/win relationships. You can learn to rejoice both for your success and the success of others. You learn you influence and are influenced by others through kindness, meekness, and love. (See *Moral Limbo, p. 10.*)

As you heal you will learn you are now safe from being completely controlled. You can be safe from helplessness because you have matured to adulthood. (See *Erikson Chart, p. 5; Parenting the Inner Child, p. 123.*)

You can recognize the power and capacity you have to act, and if someone exercises unrighteous dominion, you have power to view it from an eternal perspective. (See *Why God's Power Is Greater than Satan's, p. 289.*)

You have the ability to learn and gain inspiration that surpasses your pain. You have the ability to work on problems so continual gain and growth is experienced. For <u>no one</u> can destroy you or hurt you permanently. You can choose how to respond to the decisions of others. (See *After the Storm Comes the Rainbow, p. 311.*)

Sept. 11, 1994. I have struggled with problems between Brian and me. I have been upset almost every day for quite a while with Brian. I feel so much anger. It is almost as though I am insatiable about my problem.

I am full of anger over injustice and my inability to take away his free agency. Then I ask myself, Why do I have to be in control? How can I let go and let him lead? How can I be more selfless? I believe that 80% of the problem could be resolved through my efforts.

My husband is not a controlling man. I wanted to control him, so this was an issue for me. I had to learn to give and take control in various aspects of my life.

During childhood you were controlled and survived it. It was useful and necessary to survive the acts of another. You are a heroine to have survived.

Now as you learn and apply principles of healing, you can find peace. You can allow yourself to do what you choose. You don't have to be threatened by the choices of others. You won't be if you allow God to be in charge of eternal consequences to bring reward or punishment as He dictates.

Freedom comes as you no longer need to be in control of others. One of the greatest gifts of healing I have discovered is feeling at peace to allow others to do and learn for themselves and not feel responsible for this process.

Conclusion:
1. Being controlled by a perpetrator may result in you feeling you must be in control of every situation now.

2. God is an example to follow. He gives and He receives.

3. As you heal you will be able to give and receive. You are in control some of the time and you allow others to be in control part of the time.

PERFECTIONISM

Why do I feel like I'm never good enough?

How do I get over feeling that if people really knew me they would hate me?

Many abuse victims are broken and overworked because they are attempting to be perfect. They don't feel they are good enough--even after much work. They feel they have no worth. They feel God will not love them unless they are perfect. They must be perfect for anyone to accept them.

When I was full of pain, I heard voices within me say, *"You aren't good enough! You'll never be able to do this! No one will help you, you have to do it alone!" My voices said, "You are bad. You can't trust yourself. You aren't capable of achieving. You are guilty. No matter what you do, it won't be right. You don't even know what you are searching for."*

Trying to hide our inner voices. I believed I could not show the outside world how the voices made me feel about myself. If I did, I would surrender to what I feared most-- hopelessness. I would feel hopeless because I would have had to admit that the voices were right. I had to prove those voices wrong or change them by overcoming. I tried to make sure I didn't look like I had voices screaming that I had no worth. My house looked excellent. My family, me, my church work had to be perfect. My time had to be spent perfectly in living, in service, in sacrifice, in doing.

I was living this way because of pain. I interpreted these voices to be from God so I wanted to somehow prove to Him that I would make up for whatever I had done wrong. I would not give up on trying to prove myself to Him, then the voices might leave.

I thought everyone heard the same voices and could see I was bad and unworthy. I needed to show the world that the voices were wrong. I had to prove to everyone that I was perfect or I feared they would hate or reject me.

Trying to look okay. You want to look okay and may worry about what others think. Do you imagine people judging or mocking you? Do you feel you have a neon sign on your forehead blinking that you've been abused and have no worth? You might feel ashamed and become a perfectionist because you are trying to prove to God or to other people that you're okay. If others see you are not okay you feel despair, vulnerable, and without refuge. You feel misunderstood. (See *Feeling Misunderstood, p. 20; Shame, p. 224.*)

March 23, 1993. I need to write as a release today. I feel so frustrated, depressed and tired of trying. I feel that I am struggling in a battle without a cause, answer, or motive. I want to stop being stressed, yet I have little to be stressed about.

Brian and I live by a day timer. I have a list of things I expect myself to do. I then have the list of things I should do for my health and spiritual self, then last but truly first, I have Kati, Brian, housework and keeping the family on schedule. Today I feel I'm failing in every area. Brian has tried to help me pick up the pieces of my despair, but I don't know what I want.

I tell him I need something to get me away from the schedule and do something I enjoy. Then I can't think of anything I enjoy. When I do, I feel I can't do it when I haven't completed my list of things to do.

March 12, 1996. I want to write about something I've been struggling with for a long time. My expectations of myself must be too high and unrealistic because I seldom fulfill them. I want to have the house, myself, the children clean. I want scriptures read, meals eaten, and projects worked on. I feel stressed as though what I am working on should have already been done. I've got to find more of a balance. I've got to find peace.

The voices I heard came from within myself, and were my own abused inner children. The voices were my confused and distorted conclusions, created because of pain. (See *The Broken Inner Self, p. 4; Distorted Thinking, p. 13*.)

Many voices represented developmental stages of pain. Voices stuck in the "Initiative vs. Guilt" stage said in order to be a good girl, I must do what others said was good. Voices stuck in the "Industry vs Inferiority" stage thought I must look good enough in my accomplishments in order to be liked. While voices stuck in the "Identity vs. Role Confusion" stage told me I must impress others so they would want to be near me and I would not be left alone. (See *Erikson Chart, p. 5*.)

It takes a lot of energy to feel okay to everyone. This is especially difficult with our relationship with God because He has many commandments and rigid expectations. Life can quickly feel hopeless because there appears to be no peace in righteous living. No one lives all the ways of God perfectly at once so there is never any peace.

Why repentance isn't always the answer. Every adult needs repentance, but the little children who are crying inside didn't do anything wrong and can't repent. Consequently the voices never go away. Inner children have not acted wickedly, but feel they are bad. They need empowerment to make sense of the abuse. (See *Guilt, p. 220; Shame, p. 224.*)

Repentance does not bring the promised blessings of peace. The scriptures teach that if a sinner turns to God, he has a change of heart and no longer has a disposition to do evil. He will find peace.

If you're already trying to do what is right, you are already doing your best within the damage caused by a sinful act of another. You are not responsible for the acts of others and you cannot repent for the perpetrator's act. Repentance for daily wrongs of adulthood does not give peace to heal your childhood pain.

You may feel as though you walk in a dark and dreary state. Truly you feel as if you are looking through clouded glass. As you groan in pain in the darkness, doing all you can to receive the light, you feel God does not hear your prayer or have mercy on you. You wonder how to find God's love which will fill your soul with exceedingly great joy.

When you learn that you can partake of God's love without being perfect, then you can trade perfectionism and the voices within for peace. Then you can understand that you have worth and God's love does offer the joy promised.

As you work to understand truth and teach yourself about guilt and shame, you will be able to see your inner child as good and innocent, worthy of love from you and God. It will not matter what others believe. You will discover that you have infinite worth to God though it may not be acknowledged by others.

Conclusion

1. Inner children who are in pain from abuse feel bad and unworthy. They will tell you that you are unworthy.

2. Repentance won't bring the peace hoped for because you can't repent for sins you didn't commit.

3. The need to be perfect will diminish as you heal and rid yourself of feelings of unworthiness.

DEPRESSION

How can I get over feeling I don't care about anything?

How can I face life without drugs or antidepressants?

Many abuse victims suffer from depression. The healing process is long and intense. Healing takes a lot of energy and sometimes it doesn't seem worth the effort. Depression can result from this discouragement. Victims also suffer from depression because they fear what they feel God is urging them to do. One of the side issues of depression is that some abuse victims take drugs for relief.

Depression and fear. Depression can come from being idle or not acting on what you know you should do. You may feel depressed if you don't act on truth, or thoughts that come to you to improve your life. If you get a feeling that you should end a relationship, move out, initiate a friendship, or ask someone for help, you should act on that feeling. When you don't follow ideas from the Holy Spirit, depression results. (See *How to Heal the Inner Child, p. 132.*)

You might resist what you know you should do because you are scared. It seems too hard. You want to <u>mask</u> your feelings, not experience them. You might not follow insights because it means your adult self would have to act in spite of the fears of your inner child. (See *Adult and Inner Child Conflict, p. 119*.)

Following God's will takes courage. You must be willing to experiment on ideas that come to you to help you solve problems. You must be willing to take a step in a new direction even when you are not sure where that step will lead you. (See *Following the Direction of the Holy Spirit, p. 234*.)

When I was engaged the first time it took me awhile to recognize and follow promptings I was receiving. I wanted to please others and let them tell me what God wanted. (See *Erikson Chart–Initiative vs. Guilt, p. 5; Kohlberg Chart, p. 11*.)

Different thoughts and voices told me what to do. I was practically paralyzed because I heard so many conflicting things to do. I became depressed and afraid because I was so confused. I couldn't differentiate between the God-given messages from His Spirit, the voices inside of me, or the adversary. I didn't trust my ability to receive divine guidance.

When you doubt your strength, desire, or ability to do what you feel impressed to do, Satan steps in and darkness comes. You don't survive merely by staying alive, you survive because you are willing to thrive and put forth energy to overcome. You sacrifice the comfort of the moment for a better tomorrow.

Do the little things. There are ways to help you overcome feeling paralyzed which can help free you to act on impressions. You do something hard now so you'll be more capable or stronger later. You may start with something as simple as getting out of bed when you don't feel you can. You get out of bed one day and the next day it is easier. You learn to do one hard thing, then another. Step by step you progress and move forward.

During my engagement I felt a deep depression. The engagement came fast and I felt trapped and powerless to act. It took courage to do small acts I felt would help me. I prayed to see clearly what was happening. I prayed in great detail. My answers came while on my knees. Afterward, I couldn't differentiate answers because other voices were screaming at me. I would have to remember the answer I had received during prayer so I could move forward. While praying I got the impression to go to counseling. This was a blessing because the counselor gave me specific suggestions to follow.

One small thing I was guided to do was get some reading material on marriage. As I read the material, I discovered I didn't feel the way I should about our relationship. This gave me courage to talk to my fiancé about my concerns.

Each act strengthened me to do the next until I was able to break off the engagement. I should note here that I was not engaged to a wicked man. I simply could not feel at peace to enter this marriage relationship.

Later, when I got engaged to Brian, my husband, I immediately had doubts and fears again. I prayed to receive peace that comes only from God through His Spirit, and I was blessed with peace. Logically, there were a lot of things I didn't know, but when I knelt to ask, the peace would return. Peace is the one gift no other source can duplicate. Peace, even while feeling uncomfortable, can help us see we are being directed by God.

Sept. 20, 1991. I called my mom to tell her I was engaged to Brian. I asked her to pray for me because I was starting to feel new fears and uncertainty. Since Mom and I talked, I have been full of peace and am very happy about my decision.

Nov. 20, 1991. I feel so at peace about marrying Brian. A week from today I will marry him. I pray the spirit of God will be there. I hope I will feel at peace and full of joy. I still deal with pain from the abuse. As I spent time in prayer about this I felt that I must not hold on to the pain anymore, but give it to the Savior.

Analyze feelings to overcome depression. To write about fears lessens them. It brings them out in the open so you can look at them. Adults can think abstractly. You need to look at fears and think about the reasoning behind the fear. Fears come from the inner child's perception of the world.

The inner child is looking for people to confirm that she is safe. She wants those around her to say, "Do this. This is what is right for you." She feels she can't trust herself or her feelings. When you analyze the reasons for your fears, you start to see how your inner child is feeling. (See *Adult and Inner Child Conflict, p. 119.*)

Writing in a journal is incredibly helpful in moving you to action. Journal writing leads you to discover the many ways to overcome depression. It is a way of listening to your own feelings and understanding how to resolve your problems. Journal writing makes thoughts and feelings real giving courage to apply those thoughts and feelings. (See *Journal Writing, p. 271.*)

Depression and drugs. Because depression is difficult, many victims take drugs for relief. Taking prescription drugs can ultimately create a situation where you get stuck and can't truly heal. Drugs can mask how you are feeling. Drugs temporarily take care of the feeling of depression, but you can heal in monumental ways when you can honestly feel where you are in your life. (See *Second Sins, p. 171.*)

I took an antidepressant during my first engagement. I received an impression later to stop. Taking antidepressants affects my ability to feel impressions or recognize my own feelings. I needed to feel what I was really experiencing if I wanted to heal.

July 19, 1989. I started taking antidepressant pills this week. I felt like I needed to be less tense, serious and stressed out about life. When I look at it realistically, there is no reason to be so intense about life or to fear things. I have decided to exercise daily and take this medicine and see what happens. If it is like before, I will be doing super and feel more relaxed about life in a couple of days.

If you are taking medications, do not just go off them. Analyze why you use them and determine if you have a permanent or temporary need. Pray for understanding of what will best help you heal. Learn all you can from your doctor. Ask your doctor how long he expects you to be on the medication. Ask how he feels about you going off your medication to try coping without it.

When you follow the direction that comes from spiritual experience, you will receive ideas that may help you to be able stop prescription drugs so that you don't need antidepressants. You will be building good habits for life--not just to get you off prescriptions. Be sure you've built good, strong habits before you let go of something that has been helping you. (See *How to Heal the Inner Child, p. 132.*)

You can overcome depression. Start by acting on inspiration you receive from the Lord. There are many sources of depression. Ask Father in Heaven to guide you in discovering the source of your depression. God will guide you as you try to overcome this trial in your life.

Conclusion:

1. One way to overcome depression is to follow spiritual insight.

2. When you write in a journal, you'll find ways to heal as you analyze what you need to do.

3. God's Spirit will whisper peace as you receive inspiration. Satan cannot duplicate peace.

4. Look carefully at whether you should start or stop using medication.

FEELING I SHOULDN'T BE ANGRY

Did God allow me to experience abuse so I would be better for it?

If I get angry, won't I have to repent for it?

When you are passive, you continue to feel broken. When you think you deserve to suffer, you negate your worth. You do not <u>deserve</u> suffering. Your inner child didn't deserve abuse or suffering. She deserved nurturing, love, and trusting relationships. She deserved to be taught eternal truths. This is what God wants for <u>all</u> children, but because of the law of agency He must allow pain.

Thinking God made the abuse happen keeps you victimized. There is some truth, but it is twisted into an untruth. God did not <u>do</u> this to you. God does not inflict pain on innocent or righteous people. He sadly stands back and allows pain because of mankind's agency.

Be angry about evil. If you have not felt angry about the abuse you experienced, you are probably still feeling like a victim. Anger can be good. It helps you progress from feeling like a victim to feeling like you have self worth. Learn to make a stand against the evil that happened to you.

If you believe that you as a child deserved to be hurt and you cannot be angry about it, you sabotage your ability to progress in healing. It leaves you helpless and hopeless, feeling victimized by God himself.

Several therapists told me I had to feel angry about what happened in order to become whole. I resisted their counsel feeling expressing anger was evil or a sin. I was determined that I was not going to sin in order to heal. I couldn't imagine God telling me I was innocent of the abuse, but I would have to do things that were wrong to heal.

God is angry about evil. I felt anger was wrong and I would have to repent later if I got angry. I felt if I never got angry then I wouldn't need to repent for not forgiving the perpetrator and being angry at him for what he had done. I felt stuck. (See *Feelings about the Perpetrator, p. 44.*)

One day, pondering my dilemma, I had a flashback. I saw myself at a despairing moment experiencing painful abuse. A thought came, *Imagine the Savior standing here watching all of this happen. How does He feel?*

The answer was, "He was <u>angry</u>!" I wondered why and the thought came, *Your body is a temple. How did the Savior feel about the temple being desecrated while He was on earth? What did He do about it?*

Imagine how much our Savior cares when our body, a temple of God, is desecrated. When I realized God was not indifferent about my painful experiences, I could stand firm to cleanse the damage that was done. God was angry about my abuse. He was working passionately to help me fix the damage that was done. God does not approve of evil. His wrath is kindled against it.

It has been reassuring to discover later that other

victims of abuse were given the same inspiration about anger. Their thoughts were also turned to Christ cleansing the temple.

Anger is empowering. You have a right to be angry about the evil about which God feels angry. It is important to feel angry. The abuse happened. There is evil in the world and you experienced some of it. God is angry about wicked acts. (See *Constructive Uses of Anger, p. 39*.)

Study what God says about sins of mankind and innocent children being hurt. Stand against evil so you don't feel like a victim. Work with God and fight your war against Satan. You must stand firm against evil acts so you can work with the Savior to conquer the effects of your abuse.

Mar. 13, 1997. I am amazed at the things written in the scriptures about God's anger toward the wicked. I often feel my inner children are crying from the dust for the vengeance that God executes upon those who destroy his people. I have learned the Lord will execute vengeance and fury upon the unrepentant.

There are tons of scriptures on the subjects of judgment, vengeance, wrath, fury, wickedness. It is very healing and healthy for me to read and find that good will conquer evil. God does bless righteousness and He will not stand for wickedness. The wicked belong to Satan to be bound and spiritually destroyed. Our actions do have consequences. Good will be restored to good and evil to evil, everything in its proper order in the eternities. The righteous will conquer because of the Son of God our atoner and Redeemer.

You cannot be passive to achieve the potential for which you long. God can't work with indifference. He says, "I would thou wert cold or hot" (Rev. 3:15). As you learn how you have been affected by abuse you will want to stand up for the truth and fight against evil. God will stand with you.

Conclusion:
1. Passive feelings about your abuse keep you victimized.
2. God takes a stand against evil and you should too.

CONSTRUCTIVE USES OF ANGER
How can I overcome feelings of anger?
Is anger bad or wicked?

Anger is a feeling of wanting to gain control over one's pain. It is a firm expression of what the pain means to the person. Anger brings a feeling of power that helps overcome victimized feelings. It is a protection. It is a way to protect the primary emotion that makes you feel vulnerable.

Anger masks other emotions, so it can be considered a secondary emotion. A person usually expresses anger in order to protect feelings of intense pain or fear. Other emotions climax into anger.

Imagine you are outside and you see your toddler chasing a ball toward a busy street. You feel pain, "I could lose my baby!" You run for her, fearful she'll be hurt. You reach her just as she steps off the curb. Angry, you grab her, "You could have been killed!" Pain and fear erupt into anger.

Anger is an important part of healing. Anger helps you gain power over your own life so you no longer feel like a victim. Anger needs to be constructive to be helpful in healing. Anger is healthy if it is used productively, but it must be controlled. It needs to accomplish something. The act of destroying won't move anger into progressive healing. (See *Feeling I Shouldn't Be Angry, p. 36.*)

This is a journal entry I wrote for counseling to analyze why I was angry:

May/June 1996. I am angry because–The world is unjust. I am lonely, abandoned and full of pain. I long for good but sabotage it because of a lack of trust, a belief I don't deserve good. I feel Brian doesn't really care.

I am hurt by Brian. He is not sensitive, won't share. I can't share–I'm too vulnerable. I want him to know what I need and to help me. I so wish he would spend time with me. I wish he would be assertive, want to talk, be affectionate. I wish I didn't have to ask for things I desire and then feel unworthy to have.

I wish I wouldn't reject Brian. I wish I could spend time with Brian and tell him what I need. I wish I would communicate my feelings. I wish I wouldn't sabotage his goodness and love. I wish I would accept his love. I wish I had more faith. I wish I wasn't so angry. I wish I could change myself. I wish we weren't workaholics.

Making anger constructive. First, choose the correct focus. When you feel anger about your abuse, concentrate on the act and not the perpetrator. The perpetrator has his own complex story which is impossible to surmise.

Who knows where the perpetrator will stand before God? He could have been abused himself and doesn't know how to heal. Perhaps he is trying to heal but is acting out his own abuse. He could be mentally unstable. He could be anything! (See *Feelings about the Perpetrator, p. 44.*)

The whole of it is that what the perpetrator did was evil. When you feel anger remember –the ACTION was so wrong.

The anger goes to the act. This makes anger progressive. (See *Forgiveness, p. 47.*)

The Savior exemplified controlled anger. As in all things, the Savior set the example. You can even look to Him to see how to control anger. When Christ cleansed the temple, the first thing He felt was pain. These men were desecrating His Father's house. He showed this pain through righteous and constructive anger (see John 2:13-16).

If the Savior had not responded, it would have been like saying He agreed with what happened or He was a victim to the action. His actions were a powerful statement which showed the worth of the temple.

Anger is making a stand. It is saying what happened was wrong. Abuse is an evil act and God is not pleased it happened. He does not believe you deserved to be exploited, hurt, and broken. He is angry about it, too.

Jesus showed how He felt about the temple being desecrated. Paul said, "Know ye not that ye are the temple of God. . .If any man defile the temple of God, him shall God destroy; for the temple of God is holy, which temple ye are" (1 Cor. 3:16-17). Your body is a temple! It was desecrated! You, with God, can be angry about it.

I found it very helpful to read scriptures about God's wrath towards evil. Read scriptures about wrath, fury, and indignation to see how the Lord acts when He is angry.

Put your energy into the fight to survive. Think of your anger as if you are in a war. Don't use your energy wondering why the enemy is fighting or who is to blame for the war. Fight the war of healing and look to God to win.

Many prophets watered their pillows at night because of evil. They fought for freedom with emotion. Evil puts us into bondage. Evil is wrong! We must seek to break the chains of bondage sin brings to freedom. The righteous are to stand against it. Stand against evil with emotion.

Tell God how you feel about being abused. It was wrong! God wants you to know it was wrong for you to have been hurt. You are His child. He loves you. You didn't deserve to be hurt by another's evil act. You are beautiful.

When I was feeling angry about my abuse, I looked at a picture of the Savior and had this incredible impression: *You have always felt the perpetrator's acts would hold you back. Because of me, their acts can't hold you back, but you will hold them back because they dirtied their hands with their acts upon you. They will be held back and you will be a witness before their face always. What they did will <u>never</u> leave them unless they come unto me.*

This thought gave me hope. I felt like my destiny was in my hands and not determined by the acts of my perpetrators. I could move forward in spite of the terrible things that had happened to me.

Facing your perpetrator. Here is a way I worked through some anger. I wrote this letter to one of my perpetrators. Facing the damage of a perpetrator's acts can be healthy. Your adult self can see the perpetrator in a new light. The inner child can learn that an adult (you) will stand up to her abuser to protect her from evil. This is very healing.

Don't write, call, or visit a perpetrator expecting the abuser to apologize. Not surprisingly, this abuser has not responded to my letter. Most of the time the perpetrator will deny, accuse, or justify his behavior. Do some therapy work with a counselor before you write.

Seeing through a Glass Darkly

Dear Mr. Jones, (not real name)

I'm sure you remember me if you allow yourself. My name (maiden) is Julie Gilbert. I lived on the opposite corner from you. You sexually abused me in your apartment, barn and basement laundry room from about seven to nine years of age.

You used pornography, oral sex, and intercourse. When I was a child, I felt there was something secret and uncomfortable with the things you did. I did not know then that what you did was very wrong. You used me to fulfill your sexual desires. You hurt me!

You used my innocence, trust, sweetness and childlike self and slayed my inner peace for your own selfish pleasure. I am angry at you for caring for nothing but the moment, for having or using no self control, for caring nothing for another.

You have caused confusion, self doubt, and pain in my life. You have robbed me of deserved peace, love and an ability to see and understand sexuality in the positive ways it was meant.

I used to think that your actions and those of others like you would hold me back, but I want you to know that I will hold you back. Your actions towards me will stand as a witness against you. God will not let you walk away seemingly clean from such a filthy act. Your actions were evil and your acts on my innocence will be all over your hands, body and face.

God will not hold you blameless unless in this life you go to Him full of sorrow and confess and repent. If not, the Atonement of Christ will be void on your account, your actions will stay with you and you will suffer the pains of a damned soul. You will suffer for your own sins because you refused to come unto Christ who suffered for us all. I want you to know that at the judgment bar I will stand as a witness against you.

But if you will pour out your heart to God, confess of your doings to those in authority, that stain will be gone from you and you will be able to start on a path of your own healing and cleansing. I hope you will do this. Your actions were ugly and inexcusable.

You can repent. <u>I want you to know this.</u> That our hands may both be clean as we stand at the bar of judgment is up to our own choices. Repent or be damned.

Anger is a powerful force. Use it to stand against evil and stop feeling victimized. You will keep your anger constructive if you focus on rebuilding your life rather than retaliating towards someone who hurt you.

Conclusion:
1. Anger surfaces because of deeper emotions.
2. Constructive anger makes a stand against evil. The Savior is the perfect example of constructive anger. Study God's words concerning His wrath toward evil acts.
3. Focus your energy on healing–not on the perpetrator.
4. Abuse will not hold you back. It will hold back the perpetrator.
5. If you confront an abuser, do it for your own healing with no expectations from him.

FEELINGS ABOUT THE PERPETRATOR
How can I heal when my perpetrator won't even admit he abused me?

How can I get over being consumed by hateful feelings about the perpetrator?

Feelings about the perpetrator can make you feel shattered. You can become consumed about him to the point you focus on him and not yourself. You may spend your time wishing he would be exposed for what he is really like. You may even try to convince people what he is like. When you focus on the perpetrator, you are not focusing on your healing.

It is comforting to know that God is unhappy with those that hurt his little ones. The Lord asked Cain, "Where is Abel thy brother?" (Gen. 4:9). God knew Abel had been hurt and

44

asked Cain, "What hast thou done? the voice of thy brother's blood crieth unto me from the ground" (v. 10). Cain was cursed for his assault on his brother. God hears the prayers of His children and is aware of their suffering. He is aware of your pain.

God knows each person's heart. Your perpetrator may seem to prosper in this life, but God understands his motivation. God sees the perpetrator's actions and knows his heart.

"Not every one that saith unto me, Lord, Lord, shall enter into the kingdom of heaven; but he that doeth the will of my Father which is in heaven.

"Many will say to me in that day, Lord, Lord, have we not prophesied in thy name? and in thy name have cast out devils? and in thy name done many wonderful works?

"And then will I profess unto them, I never knew you: depart from me, ye that work iniquity" (Matt. 7:21-23).

God knows that outward actions do not always match the heart. The goal in life is not to do lots of good things, it is to become like God. A perpetrator may be talented, "religious," and kind to others; but this may only be a way to cover evil in his life. It is difficult to ever tell.

If the person does good, it is still good. Good acts may not benefit the perpetrator on judgment day because the appearance of good does not erase evil, only repentance can do that. You don't have to worry about the perpetrator's motives when he does good. God knows the heart of every person.

At times the Holy Ghost will help by manifesting someone's intents, but other times you simply will not know. What the person did is between him and God. Separate the perpetrator from the abuse. "Vengeance is mine; I will repay, saith the Lord" (Rom. 12:19).

Repeatedly I dreamed of hot fudge being poured over mud. I saw an ice cream scoop of mud on a beautiful plate with hot fudge poured generously on top. Who would know that this wasn't the best sundae in the world? God knows, and thus no unclean thing can enter the kingdom of God no matter how good it looks.

God will deal justly with each of his children. God does not tell perpetrators or offenders He will stop them from abusing. He says there will be serious consequences for those that hurt the little children. God will chastise and deal justly with the perpetrator.

"But whoso shall offend one of these little ones which believe in me, it were better for him that a millstone were hanged about his neck, and that he were drowned in the depth of the sea" (Matt. 18:6).

Focus on healing rather than on the perpetrator. If you work to focus on the evil act of the abuser and not on the abuser as evil, you can work through healing more directly. If you wait for the perpetrator to change in order to heal, you are stuck–angry, full of pain and unable to move forward. You are responsible for your own actions, not the perpetrator's actions.

To focus on the abuser is like focusing on Satan saying, "When he changes and doesn't tempt me, then I'll be happy." This only robs you. Satan won't change and he wants you to be miserable like he is. Your perpetrator may never change and he may want you to be miserable, too. You give control to others when your healing is conditional on their actions. Leave the perpetrator with God, focus on the act so you can heal from being miserable.

You were wronged when you were abused. Your

46

perpetrator sinned in abusing you. Find comfort in the knowledge that God is just and He knows His children. He will deal justly with your perpetrator, it is not your problem. Work to heal from your pain and find the peace and joy you deserve.

Conclusion:

1. Perpetrators have sinned in hurting little children.

2. Perpetrators do good acts as well as bad ones. Let God judge them.

3. Don't focus on the perpetrator. Work on healing whether or not the perpetrator changes.

4. Satan and those who do evil acts want others to be miserable like they are.

5. Don't give control to others. Focus on healing to be free of misery.

FORGIVENESS

How can I forgive someone who betrayed me?
Do I have to forgive before I can heal?

Forgiveness may seem to be a difficult part of healing. You may struggle if you are counseled to first forgive before you will heal. When you focus on healing, forgiveness can be a natural result. When you try to force forgiveness at the beginning of healing, you may minimize or bury the abuse experience instead--ignoring it or putting it behind you without working through it.

It is difficult to expect forgiveness at the beginning or middle of healing. The best thing to do is actively focus on what it takes to heal. Then when all the layers of pain are peeled away, you can look at what is left. I found peace was left.

Focus on healing. Forgiveness came naturally because I learned to focus my energy on <u>what</u> happened, not <u>who</u> abused me. Focus on the act. The <u>act</u> was wrong.

You do not need to understand the perpetrator or his motivation. You must face and deal with how the act affected you. You must work through your feelings of pain and sorrow because of the acts of sin. To focus on <u>what</u> was done and not <u>who</u> did it frees you from needing to repent later for being unforgiving. (See *Feelings about the Perpetrator, p. 44.*)

When you do not forgive, you judge another person. You decide that person has done something so wrong he cannot be forgiven. You stand in God's place as a judge. Forgiveness means you leave judgment to God. God understands all.

As I healed, I discovered a love toward my grandfather who abused me. I feel he too had been abused. Perhaps his was a dual problem of being a victim and a perpetrator. I hope he is proud of me for breaking the bonds of pain he never had the courage to face.

Anger and forgiveness. You will probably feel anger during your healing process. You might wonder if you should suppress it. It was difficult for me to get angry because I wanted to know--why anger? why blame? If I chose to be angry, I felt I would commit sin in the healing process and would have to repent later for the anger. The process that was supposed to heal me wasn't supposed to damage me at the same time. (See *Feeling I Shouldn't Be Angry, p. 36.*)

I had to learn that anger was useful because being hurt by another person was wrong. I learned that being angry could be a righteous act of standing against evil. It is important to stand up to evil acts. God is angry because of unrepentant sinful acts. Be angry about the abuse, but don't focus on the perpetrator. (See *Constructive Uses of Anger, p. 39.*)

An ancient story. Long ago there was a father who talked to each of his sons before he died. One of the father's youngest sons had been dealt with abusively by some older brothers and the father taught this son how to deal with the past abusiveness of his brothers.

The son needed to know God's compassion encompassed his pain. The father taught his son his afflictions would be a blessing, telling the son that God would consecrate his afflictions for his gain.

The father did not preach that this son was responsible to forgive his brothers. He did not attack or blame the brothers. The father focused on the fact that the actions of the brothers had caused pain.

The son was not asked to live with the abusive brothers, but was instructed to dwell safely with a kindly older brother. As the abused son concentrated on what was good and safe, he was able to leave the pain behind.

As this young son eventually learned to stand firmly against evil, this resulted in strength of character as he came to know God. He became a leader to others. He taught people who had been hurt and who were hurting others. I believe forgiveness came naturally for him as he focused on what to do to overcome the abusive acts of his brothers.

Revenge and retaliation. Learning to forgive means refraining from retaliation, vengeance, and malice. We don't ask an eye for an eye or a tooth for a tooth. Forgiveness is allowing time during the healing process so God can give us spiritual understanding and peace. Forgiveness is natural if we seek God's guidance during healing.

This does not mean we can't ask, "Why?" or "How

could someone do this?" You will want to ask, "How am I supposed to respond to this situation now?" It is important to explore questions like these in the process of healing.

Avoid thoughts such as, "I hate him!" or "I'll show him!" When you hear yourself saying, "I'll never forgive him," or "I'll get back at him," seek God's help to soften your heart. Give the pain and judgment to God.

You may feel an obligation to protect others from being wounded and so you may have to deal with legal and church action as you resolve your problems. These authorities can help guide the perpetrator to healing and repentance. As you turn information to authorities, it is important to view this as an act of mercy that allows the perpetrator to face his life, change and repent, and put it in order.

Forgiveness is:
- Judging the action, not the person's state of mind or spirit.
- Allowing God to judge the perpetrator.
- Focusing on how the pain affects you and working through it with the help of God.
- Enabling the perpetrator to take responsibility for his acts through proper authority and law.
- Standing before God accountable for your own acts, not damning or excusing yourself because of the acts of others.

Forgiveness is not:
- Seeking revenge.
- Trusting the perpetrator in situations where you or he is vulnerable.
- Protecting the perpetrator from consequences.
- Pretending acts are okay when they are not, saying the perpetrator didn't really hurt you.
- Trying to forget the whole thing, saying it never happened.

Focusing on the perpetrator robs you of healing. In your work to heal, remember to concentrate on yourself and not the perpetrator. You will discover one of the miracles of forgiveness is that when you are actively involved in keeping the commandments and working through healing, forgiveness will usually take care of itself.

Conclusion:

1. When you are more angry at a person than you are at their actions, you are judging the person.

2. You aid your healing when you work through your pain rather than focus on the perpetrator.

3. You can be angry about sinful acts without being revengeful toward the perpetrator.

4. When you focus on healing from abuse, forgiveness usually follows.

CHAPTER TWO

THE GLASS MAGNIFYING THE INNER SOUL

"And the Lord said. . . This day will I begin to magnify thee in the sight of all Israel, that they may know that, as I was with Moses, so I will be with thee" (Joshua 3:7).

Moses was a man who had limitations of speech and a great work to do despite his limitations. God provided help so Moses could do God's work. Moses' help came in the form of his brother, Aaron. By providing the help for which Moses asked, Moses was magnified to become a deliverer. With Aaron's help, Moses' abilities were expanded and he accomplished God's will.

God's will is to deliver your inner children. He has given you the means to lead them to deliverance. As you prayerfully choose your course of healing, be sure to utilize the strengths God has gifted to others to help guide your course. Your path to deliverance will be smoother if you use the tested truths others have successfully used to aid in your liberation. Open your eyes to those who have found answers linking them to truth.

Then, as Moses led those in bondage to the promised land, your inner children will be delivered as you lead them to God's promised peace within.

RECOGNIZING SIGNS OF ABUSE

How will I be able to tell if someone has been abused?

What should I look for if I'm wondering if someone has been abused?

When people have been through trauma, they struggle with many similar problems. An abuse victim is not going to have all the signs listed below. Someone who is <u>not</u> an abuse victim may show many of these signs when struggling with life. These are merely a guide to help you know some things you might want to look for.

- Low self-esteem. She feels inferior to others. She often compares herself unfavorably with others. She searches to be accepted by others, but even when she is given a compliment, she is unable to accept it. (See *Loss of Identity as a Follower of Christ, p. 212*.)

- She comments on injustice and feels anger toward rules or set programs. (See *Kohlberg Chart, p. 11*.)

- She talks about feeling or being different. (See *Feeling Misunderstood, p. 20*.)

- She suffers from extreme emotional lows. She seems unable to have balance in her life. (See *Depression, p. 31*.)

- She has issues about men. She feels the other gender has complete dominance. (See *Control Issues, p. 23; Feelings about the Perpetrator, p. 44*.)

- She often wants to avoid certain situations. She may hate to be in crowds or may avoid a situation that reminds her consciously or unconsciously of the abuse. (See *The Broken Inner Self, p. 4*.)

- She seems unable to enjoy the simple things of life. (See *Adult and Inner Child Conflict, p. 119.*)

- She struggles with maintaining healthy relationships. She may have experienced multiple divorces. She destroys dating relationships. She struggles with close lasting friendships. She may choose to isolate herself from others. (See *Control Issues, p. 23; Sexual Boundaries, p. 180.*)

- She feels misunderstood in conversations—especially on religious or moral subjects. (See *Feeling Misunderstood, p. 20.*)

- She keeps her life private and even secretive because she feels that if others knew about the abuse they would judge, reject, or ostracize her. (See *Feeling Misunderstood, p. 20.*)

- She feels no one cares what happens to her. She feels she is unimportant to others and they would be better off without her. (See: *Nurturing–Learning to Help Yourself, p. 147.*)

- She may experience nightmares and restless sleeping patterns. (See *Recovering Memories through Dreams, p. 95.*)

- She may be unable to make decisions in stressful circumstances. (See *The Broken Inner Self, p. 4.*)

- She may be very compulsive. She may be showing that no one will ever control her again. Some signs of compulsive-ness are a perfectly clean home or a perfect looking family. (See *Perfectionism, p. 27.*)

- At the other extreme, she may still play the role of a victim and be very passive. (See *Control Issues, p. 23.*)

- She may punish or hurt herself. You might see scars on her arms. She may restrict her eating habits excessively or not allow herself to enjoy good things in life like family or religious activities. She feels she doesn't deserve anything good. (See *Strengthening against Damaging Cycles, p. 260.*)

- She may struggle with anxiety. (See *The Broken Inner Self, p. 4; First-Time Flashbacks, p. 98.*)

- She may appear guilt ridden. (See *Guilt, p. 220.*)

- She may seem numb, like she is trying to avoid any emotion. (See *Understanding Suffering, p. 293.*)

- She may show anger at inappropriate times and in inappropriate ways. (See *The Broken Inner Self, p. 4.*)

While these signs may not be all inclusive, they will give you an idea of what to look for. When you see several of these signs, investigate further because something is going on. Quite probably you will find a victim of abuse.

When you find an opportunity to talk, share your observations then ask, "What has caused you to see yourself in this distorted way?" Or you might ask, "What kind of trauma or problem would cause this trial?"

Listen as the person shares why she thinks she is struggling. If the answer she shares sounds trivial or doesn't match up, reply, "I am learning that current problems can stem back to our earliest years as a child. What was childhood like for you?"

This kind of sharing may open the door for the person to begin to discover the root of a lot of her daily problems. It may bless her life with the opportunity to connect her childhood to the present, to feel accepted and invited to seek healing. Prayerfully doing this can bless lives.

Many will have behaviors on this list which stem from difficulties other than sexual abuse. You can be a support to others regardless of their burden. Some abuse victims may not tell you about their abuse for a long time. Others may be at a point to willingly share because of your concern. Regardless of how or when they share, recognize that those who struggle through daily life feel alone. If they allow themselves to be helped, you could be a true friend.

WILL I EVER HEAL?

Even if I am willing to heal, will I ever feel whole again?

Is it possible to heal completely?

You may ask yourself, "Will I ever heal completely? Will the effects of abuse always be a stumbling block in my life? You may see your pain as a deep wound that needs to be lanced. You doctor it and care for it and eventually it heals, but there is always a scar.

I believe that the damage from trauma is more aptly compared to breaking your leg. You can leave the leg alone, broken, and get around the best you can. You might use crutches or drag the leg behind you. When you decide you want to be whole, you reset the leg so it can heal correctly. One day you will run again if you work to heal it completely through the proper attention. You need not always be scarred. (See *Should I Go to Therapy? p. 77.*)

Look to good examples. I once asked a lady I admired what she did to become such a good woman. She said she studied great women (women in the scriptures, mothers, honorable women from history). She tried to emulate the great qualities of exemplary ladies around her. She did not focus on bad examples.

What do you want to be? Forget about talking and concentrating on what you don't want. Focus on what you desire.

Great women are those who live actively, passionately, and prayerfully. They believe good will come from the sacrifice, love, and patience they exhibit. All great women have overcome some obstacle in their path. Let good examples help you believe that somehow you can overcome your obstacles and stand with them. You can do it. Believe it!

Look to the Savior. Of course your best example is the Savior. He is not simply a good example, He is your Redeemer. He can heal you completely. Jesus has power to heal any sickness or malady. "And Jesus went about all Galilee, . . . healing all manner of sickness and all manner of disease among the people" (Matt. 4:23).

You are required to actively do all you can to help it happen. You cannot heal passively. You must courageously and actively apply healthy habits and thinking in your life. You must look to the Savior rather than focus on your wounds. (See *Willingness to Heal, p. 58.*)

You may feel like the woman who "having an issue of blood twelve years, which had spent all her living upon physicians, neither could be healed of any" (Luke 8:43). She had spent time and money trying to heal, but she was ultimately made whole through the healing power of the Savior.

If you believe in the redemption of Christ you can be healed. You can heal completely. You can have a wonderful life. The Savior is the way to find that healing.

Conclusion:

1. Look to good examples and emulate them.

2. Actively do all you can do to heal, then trust the Savior to do the rest.

3. You can heal completely from abuse.

WILLINGNESS TO HEAL

I'm doing okay, why should I try and change my life?

How can I believe Christ will heal me?

When a person is sick, it is logical to do whatever needs to be done to get well. Sometimes, however, people don't get the help they need. Imagine a woman has chronic pain. She could go to the doctor and see what is wrong, but there are lots of reasons why she may not.

Maybe she doesn't like doctors or doesn't believe doctors can help. She may have had a bad experience with a doctor and so seeing one seems like part of the problem rather than part of the cure. Maybe she would rather endure the known pain than risk new unknown pain caused by probing, experimenting, or surgery.

She may even avoid the doctor fearing she has an incurable disease. She thinks she'd rather not know for sure. She thinks if she ignores the pain, it will go away. She may avoid the doctor thinking the pain is in her head and the doctor will tell her she is crazy.

Each of these fears and doubts may keep a person from seeking help. But each person must make a decision about whether to heal and how to go about it. We are in charge of our healing.

Choose to leave bondage. The Israelites offer an example of people who were given a choice of leaving their known life in bondage for a new, unknown life in freedom.

The Israelites were in bondage through no fault of their own. During the time of Joseph their ancestors had been invited to live in Egypt, but now they were slaves. The Egyptians "made their lives bitter with hard bondage, in morter, and in brick, and in all manner of service in the field: all their service, wherein they made them serve, was with rigour" (Ex. 1:14).

But God had not forgotten His children. "And I have also heard the groaning of the children of Israel, whom the Egyptians keep in bondage; and I have remembered my covenant" (Ex. 6:5).

God hears the cries of those who suffer. His heart must break for those who suffer innocently because of the wickedness of others. He remembers and keeps the covenants He makes with His children.

God offered deliverance to the children of Israel through His prophet Moses. A lot of the Israelites did not want to leave bondage for fear of the unknown. They were comfortable even though they were miserable. They probably wanted to know exactly how long the journey would take, where they would get food, how Moses would get them across the Red Sea. They wanted to know the details before they would move forward.

Deliverance comes with a price. Moses was asking them to stretch. He was delivering them, but it came with a price. The Israelites had to willingly follow Moses out of bondage in order to be delivered.

Deliverance comes by actively learning, stretching, and taking risks. You can't progress in your life when you are totally comfortable. I used to think I would stop being uncomfortable when I healed, but that was not the case. Being uncomfortable is a part of life. The Lord continues to ask us to grow which means being uncomfortable and taking risks.

During their years in the wilderness, the Israelites were faced with whether or not they would heal:

"And the Lord sent fiery [poisonous] serpents among the people, and they bit the people; and much people of Israel died.

"And Moses made a serpent of brass, and put it upon a pole, and it came to pass, that if a serpent had bitten any man, when he beheld the serpent of brass, he lived" (Num. 21:6, 9).

Not all of the Israelites chose to look to the brass serpent. Why? They probably didn't look because they did not believe that it would heal them. The Israelites seem so foolish, but you may make the same mistake if you do not look to Christ because you don't believe He will heal you.

Another possible reason the Israelites did not look was because of the simplicity of the solution. They didn't believe such an easy solution could have profound results. The Savior will ask you to do simple things you <u>can</u> do to heal. As you learn God's word you need to apply simple gospel truth.

You can apply what you are able, then add more later. It is too heavy to apply everything at the beginning. God has given light and truth to many and these truths are available today. As you learn and apply truth, looking to the Savior to live, He in turn will direct your path leading you to your deliverance.

Deliverance comes through the Savior. After I learned I had been abused, I realized I could only heal by looking to the Savior. If the children of Israel had not known they were bitten by something poisonous, they would not have been responsible to find a way to be healed. But once they knew they had been bitten, Moses guided them to look at his staff which was a symbol of looking to the Savior. Ultimately, it is only through Christ we completely heal. (See *Will I Ever Heal? p. 56.*)

Just as Moses lifted up the brazen serpent in the wilderness and those who looked were healed, those who look to the Son of God with faith, having a contrite spirit, might live as well. There is no other name given under heaven but Jesus Christ, whereby man can be saved.

How do we look to the Savior? The Israelites had to do two things to be healed--turn their head and cast their eyes upward to the serpent on the staff. If they did this, they would heal. God was not asking them to stand up to walk and go to touch the staff. He didn't ask them to do something they couldn't do. They were bitten by a poisonous snake. God asked them simply to show faith in Him by looking to Him.

There are ways you can show faith in order to spiritually live. These will help you to heal and invite the Savior to take your pain:

• Recognize and follow the direction of God's Holy Spirit. (See *Following the Direction of the Holy Spirit, p. 234.*)
• Learn truth by reading God's word and soliciting His guidance.
• Write in a journal to analyze your feelings and give yourself direction. (See *Journal Writing, p. 271.*)
• Work with your inner child, nurture her, love her, teach her, and show her light and truths learned. (See *Parenting the Inner Child, p. 123.*)

At times I wondered how deep I had to dig, how far I would have to reach within myself to find answers. The answers are there. God loves you. He wants you to overcome and become like Him. You can't do that without going through some of what He did. I feel it an honor from God to have a trial that would stretch my soul so that I might have even a taste of what the Savior suffered.

July 2, 1996. I believe that as we begin our lives each one starts out with enthusiasm and optimism,

61

determined and believing we can conquer anything. Then comes the day when we may experience shock at the cross we are asked to bear.

The Savior, too, may not have expected His burden to feel so heavy. As He knelt in the garden suffering for us He said, "Let this cup pass from me, nevertheless thy will be done." God's will was done. Jesus stayed and suffered even though it meant excruciating pain. An angel was sent to minister unto Him. There have been or will be times in each of our lives when we must choose whether we stay and endure to the end or try to escape pain.

Those who followed Moses through the wilderness had to become physically and emotionally strong to make it to the chosen land. You can make it to the chosen land, too. You can choose to be strong. You are elect. You are chosen. The Savior considered you worth His great suffering. He does not ask you to do what you cannot. He asks you to do what He knows you can do and no more.

Peter said, "Blessed be the God and Father of our Lord Jesus Christ, which according to his abundant mercy hath begotten us again unto a lively hope by the resurrection of Jesus Christ from the dead.

"To an inheritance incorruptible, and undefiled, and that fadeth not away, reserved in heaven for you" (1 Peter 1: 3-4).

Come to Christ. Honestly bring all of you--the pain and confusion of your inner child. Bring your whole self to Him and let His words carry you beyond this vale of sorrow into a far better land of promise.

Conclusion:
1. You are in charge of your healing and must actively work to heal.

2. Your healing will come through the Savior.
3. Small acts of faith will lead you to healing.

DELIVERANCE IS A PROCESS

Why doesn't God just free me from my pain?
What can I do to be delivered?

Anyone in pain hopes for deliverance, longing to be out of pain enjoying peace. You may wonder why Christ doesn't simply heal you. He healed the blind and the lame. Why doesn't He make you whole?

One time when I was feeling full of pain and despair, I saw a picture of Christ healing a blind man and thought, *There must be something wrong with me. I must have no faith. If I had real faith, I would be healed. Why am I unworthy to be healed? When will I have enough faith?* Then the thought came, *You do have faith, but your healing will come after all you can do. There is so much I want you to learn.*

Use the process of healing for learning and growth. You deserve to be healed, but you are expected to overcome hardships so you will grow and stretch, "For precept must be upon precept, precept upon precept; line upon line, line upon line; here a little, and there a little" (Isaiah 28:10).

Even the Savior, innocent of sin, had to suffer. He asked, "Let this cup pass from me" (Matt. 26:39). Imagine the consequences if the Father had replied, "You don't deserve this pain. You are innocent. Let the cup pass." What would have happened to the Savior? What would have happened to all of us? The entire plan of salvation would have been thwarted.

You don't want to lose out on attaining everlasting life. The abuse was all bad. You don't want to miss out on the healing which will be all good. I honestly didn't want the Savior to take all my pain without effort from me. This would rob me of lasting growth. I did not want to be robbed of one bit of the strength that could be achieved from learning to be like the Savior. I would go through the pain, vast and intense as it might be, if God thought I could handle it.

The perpetrator could have perpetrated on anyone, but God let agency take its course and knew I could gain from healing from someone else's evil acts. I wanted to gain whatever God believed I could learn by experiencing the abuse.

Deliverance comes a step at a time. It would be nice to be made whole immediately, but deliverance often happens with small steps. Jesus healed the blind man from Bethsaida in increments.

"And he took the blind man by the hand, and led him out of the town; and when he had spit on his eyes, and put his hands upon him, he asked him if he saw ought.

"And he looked up, and said, I see men as trees, walking.

"After that he put his hands again upon his eyes, and made him look up: and he was restored, and saw every man clearly" (Mark 8:23-25).

Your healing, too, will most likely come step by step. Healing comes through small and simple things. When you are in pain you want some big event to deliver you. The tiny things you will be prompted to do will lead to big events. Actions that may seem very insignificant may lead to healing. By small and simple things great things will be brought to pass.

Following promptings from the Holy Ghost will lead you to do small things that will help you to heal. Little things can be like calling a friend you think of when you are hurting, going to see someone, or working to develop a positive new habit.

Opening the Bible and reading when the idea comes to mind is a small thing that can lead to something big. Each small idea, if acted upon, will lead to another idea and another until you see big results. Every small act can be a stepping stone to healing.

Ask for confirmation that you are making progress. When each of these "little things" happens, you can receive assurance that these are good. God will confirm it if you ask. It is not evil to ask for a confirmation of choosing the right path; this is not seeking a sign. Sign seekers want to know before they act. Confirmation is a gift given after you show faith by acting.

You may not see the confirmation or recognize it if you don't ask because of your anxiety and inner chaos. When you ask for direction, then feel and see a confirmation of approval, it helps weed out the inner chaos. You then can learn to distinguish chaos and inner voices from the still small voice of the Holy Ghost. This can bring calming and strengthening--a feeling of sanity.

Like the Savior, you must suffer to allow for progress. There is opposition in all things. If the abuse was all bad, you don't want to be robbed of the incomprehensible good that will come from working through your pain to heal. Then peace will replace your pain and through your Great Deliverer, Jesus Christ, you will be delivered from Satan's influence and the acts of abuse.

Conclusion
1. The process of deliverance is important for growth.
2. Progress often comes in small steps.
3. You can receive a confirmation that the steps you are taking are good.

THE SUREST PATH TO HEALING

How can I find a safe direction in my healing?
Church is painful for me. Why should I cling to it?

No one wants to be in pain, but you cannot avoid it
when you try to heal. You must seek for the most effective way
to heal. The more directly you heal, the sooner you can feel
peace. It is through the Savior you will heal most effectively. I
believe you can actually shorten the road to healing and apply
the teachings of the Savior by implementing these suggestions
with therapy.

Work to receive guidance from God. Listen for the
whispering of God's Spirit and follow those thoughts. Put your
trust in that Spirit which leads you to do good. Pray to learn
God's will for you. (See *Prayer, p. 247; Following the Direction of
the Holy Spirit, p. 234.*)

Be connected with Christ's gospel. Your church
should be an ally in healing. The Savior's gospel is good and
gives purpose. The church is the vehicle that carries the gospel.
Sometimes it may seem that the vehicle isn't running well, or
something is missing. Maybe your seat is very uncomfortable
with springs poking you in the back. But the Savior's word is
the vehicle that is going to help you return to God--so stay in
the vehicle.

From your seat you may not have the best view to see
all God wants to show you to help you get back to Him. But
for now you need to do what you can with what you have.
Don't give up because you are uncomfortable, lack a good
view, or are in pain because of the bumps. Hold onto the truths
with which the Holy Spirit guides you. If you feel misunderstood, remember you will receive great rewards if you endure.
(See *Feeling Misunderstood, p. 20.*)

Work with your church leader. During the process of healing, there will be times you will work closely with your religious leader. Pray for your leader so you can accomplish what is needed. Remember your clergyman desires to administer God's work. He can receive direction from God to guide people to God.

The church leader is not God. He is not all-knowing. He has his own mortal package. He may not know everything about finances or disciplining children. He may know very little about sexual abuse. Don't expect him to understand you or know how you can heal. Because of abandonment issues, when you are trying to heal you sometimes desperately look for people to help you. You may want your leader to know everything. (See *No One Will Save Me; Where Is My Savior? p. 205.*)

God has given revelation and knowledge in areas of physical and mental health. To ask your leader how you can heal is unfair; it is like asking him to help you get better when you need heart surgery. A heart surgeon is a better source for that problem just as a therapist will be a better source for helping you heal from abuse.

Your pastor is essential to help and support you spiritually. He can help you understand religious issues. Following his humble heartfelt counsel will bless your life.

Pray that you and your leader can work together to accomplish whatever will help you move forward to heal within the safety of the gospel. Seek peace of heart if your leader doesn't fulfill your needs. There will be many who will be there to help you heal. He is only one.

Feeling unworthy to attend church. One of your challenges in attending church may be getting to the point where you feel worthy to go. Seek to openly communicate with your church leader. Remember abilities never seem to match desire.

Trust that the leader might see the intent of your heart especially if you struggle with "second sins." (See *Second Sins, p. 171.*)

Show gratitude every step of the way. God gives us so much more than we can comprehend. As you show gratitude for what God has given, He will give you more. (See *Gratitude, p. 280.*)

The Savior wants you to heal safely and completely within the gospel. He has experienced all the suffering for your pain. As you seek His teachings and draw close to Him, He will show you the surest path to healing.

Conclusion:

1. The teachings of the Savior will enable you to heal more quickly.

2. You need to discover God's will for you, then do what He asks.

3. Work to make your church and church leaders your allies as you heal.

4. As you show gratitude for each blessing given, God will add more blessings.

WHAT MEN NEED TO DO TO HEAL
Why do men resist help?
How does abuse affect a man's view of sexuality?

There are many more men who suffer from abuse than are helped. Very few men seek healing though statistics say approximately one in four is abused. Why? First of all, some men who experience abuse may not even realize they have experienced abuse. Secondly, the shame of abuse attacks their identity as a capable male.

Being a victim attacks a man's innate role as a

protector. It threatens his ability to lead, solve problems, and be a source of strength to others. Sadly, society accepts men as perpetrators more readily than it accepts them as victims.

Men struggle in a society that sabotages their ability to share feelings and dreams. Men are expected to be masculine which is interpreted as being logical and unfeeling. Society feeds into this belief about men.

Men and pain. Do men hold pain inside more than women? Yes. Men feel they are not allowed to feel pain. They feel they must fix other people's problems.

Are men more vulnerable to acting out their pain? Yes, because pain will come out somehow. If a man won't ask for help or talk about his pain, it will come out negatively. Men may want to heal alone, but they can't.

How do men act out their pain? Some become perpetrators, some become depressed. Some suffer from low self-esteem and do not believe in themselves. Others compensate by becoming overachievers. Some become very controlling.

Men act much like women, but their pain is often held in longer. They don't call for help until their pain is more out of proportion. Men are often suicidal when they finally ask for help. They wait until they have absolutely no other options.

Men in the scriptures showed emotion. Men are more logical in their healing than women. Once they have talked about an issue, they don't want to talk about it any more. They want to progress to a new issue, always moving forward.

The relationship between Moses and Aaron shows an example of great men of the scriptures who shared feelings of pain and joy. They cried together, rejoiced together, suffered together, and supported each other through their trials. Knowing they were there for each other, and had a God who loved them, helped them move forward and accomplish great works. Here is one example of their cooperative help:

"And Moses said unto Joshua, Choose us out men, and go out, fight with Amalek: tomorrow I will stand on the top of the hill with the rod of God in mine hand.

"So Joshua did as Moses had said, and fought with Amalek: and Moses, Aaron, and Hur went up to the top of the hill.

"And it came to pass when Moses held up his hand, that Israel prevailed: and when he let down his hand, Amalek prevailed.

"But Moses' hands were heavy; . . . and Aaron and Hur stayed up his hands, the one on the one side, and the other on the other side; and his hands were steady until the going down of the sun" (Ex. 17: 9-12).

Counsel from therapists. Two male therapists shared some valuable insights about male victims. One said that the most helpful scripture to help men heal is, "Jesus wept" (John 11:35). It is good for men to feel emotion. If Jesus can feel, so can other men. They must feel to be able to heal. Emotions are God-given and it is good to feel them.

The other therapist suggested men remember, "Wise men seek wise counsel." Because men view themselves as protectors, they find it difficult to seek help. However, when men see that there is a need, a problem, a pain, there is wisdom in seeking capable, experienced people who can offer guidance. These people can lead them to sources to learn and apply necessary truths.

How men view sexuality. The greatest God-given difference between men and women is their sexuality--how they view it and how they function in the sexual act. For men sexuality is healing most of the time even when they have been hurt by sexuality. For women, nurturing without sexuality is most healing, even when they have not been hurt by sexuality.

Dec. 5, 1993. My relationship with Brian lacks intimacy. We need time to get close to each other. He struggles to show affection. I struggle with sex. This leaves both of us feeling unloved. It breaks down real closeness with depth of understanding toward each other.

Because many men heal with sexuality, they may be confused by the need for help with it. It is the way sexuality is governed and viewed that is the concern. It is how others are treated by their misunderstood sexuality that needs to be healed. Men's healing will bless them to become whole and Christlike so they can righteously govern those around them.

In most aspects male survivors heal the same way as female survivors. Men and women are both damaged from abuse. Both have the same broad spectrum of issues from which to heal. Men, too, are broken from being victimized. Of course, both need the Savior's Atonement to heal completely. There is no other way or name given under heaven whereby man can be saved in the kingdom of God. This is the doctrine of Christ .

Conclusion:

1. Men must deal not only with their abuse, but also with how society views men who have been abused.

2. Men cannot heal alone.

3. Men need to show emotion.

4. Men and women are different in how they view sexuality. Men find healing in sexuality, while women heal through nurturing.

HELPING OTHERS

What if I try to be a friend to an abuse victim and she starts to depend on me all the time?

What if my friend wants to tell me lots of things I don't want to hear?

If you are reading this section, you may be worried about a friend, relative, or neighbor that is struggling. You may be a church leader who wants to know how to help someone under your stewardship. You may not even know that the person has been abused, but you see suffering and you want to help. You are to be commended.

Bearing one another's burdens. You act as a disciple of Christ when you are willing to bear one another's burdens, mourn with those that mourn, and comfort those that stand in need of comfort. As a follower of Christ, you have the privilege of suffering with others.

It takes a spiritually mature person to be like the Savior and willingly suffer with another. Reaching out to someone means taking a risk and leaving your comfort zone so that you are in a position or attitude to bear someone else's burden.

It should be reassuring to know that while you should nurture those that need it, you are not responsible to solve their problems. Your genuine love and concern helps to ease their burden. In a real and tangible way you can help carry those who need to be lifted.

You can assist in deliverance. Isaiah wrote, "They shall bring thy sons in their arms, and thy daughters shall be carried upon their shoulders.

"And kings shall be thy nursing fathers, and their queens thy nursing mothers" (Isa. 49:22-23).

72

You can carry individuals who need your help and assist them in their deliverance. People who have experienced abuse need to be spiritually and emotionally carried upon the shoulders of others. Those who follow inspiration to lift and love can carry others with great burdens. The Savior will use your hands to help others if you give them to Him to use.

Most of the time when people are blessed and their suffering is eased, it is through other people. God prompts and directs people to serve others in answer to prayer. God uses willing people to help meet the needs of His children.

God's children have a responsibility to build His kingdom. Many times you might look at the pain of the world and feel helpless. You feel like turning away from it so it won't cause you pain. You feel you can't do anything.

Ultimately the Savior heals all pain. He has suffered for all suffering. You do not have to feel helpless about the pain in the world. You love others and the Savior does the healing.

God needs His people to strengthen others so they may become strong enough to overcome their internal pain. You can look for ways to assist God to help others ease their pain and look to our Savior for His atoning love that conquers pain.

Conclusion:

1. Followers of Christ reach out to others and help them.

2. You do not need to solve someone else's problems. You will be most helpful when you love and lift others.

3. Healing comes through the Savior, but the Savior will use you to meet the needs of others.

HOW DO I HELP?

*How can I help someone through abuse when I
don't know much about abuse and I don't have much time?
What if I give poor counsel and ruin someone's life?*

Many good people want to help others but are not sure
what to do. They feel because they do not know much about
abuse they cannot effectively assist an abuse victim. This section will give you practical suggestions about helping. Most of
the following suggestions, while written for helping abuse
victims, will also apply to other situations where you are
empathizing with someone in pain.

Listen. Sometimes you do the greatest good when you
don't say anything! Listen to the words and the emotion under-
lying what you hear. Listen for what is not said. Listen for the
Holy Spirit to help you know how to respond if you feel you are
to respond. You may find that sometimes the most healing thing
you can do is to simply cry together.

Give hope, not advice. When appropriate, share
your testimony that you know God cares and the Savior
conquered pain. Teach that we are here to learn to love like the
Father and his Son. Tell your friend you believe in her and help
her to know the goodness you see in her.

Check back later. Remember the story of the Good
Samaritan? The Good Samaritan helped an injured man. He
shared some of his time, money, and energy. Then he turned
the injured man over to the inn keeper. He contacted the man
later to check on his needs (see Luke 10:25-37).

You can do the same. Call your friend and ask how
she is doing. How did she do with the challenge she had? Tell

her you've been thinking of her. Tell her you've been praying for her.

When you help, you aren't expected to be <u>consumed</u>. Be aware though that your friend has experienced abandonment and you will need to earn her trust. Give what you can give now, and be committed to give what you can later. Helping can mean being there for a little while to follow through on seeing the person do better, receive strength and go forward.

You help a person with emotional pain regain trust when you offer extended caring. Abuse victims do not heal with quick fixes, so if you come in for a moment to help, then make no contact later, the victim feels abandoned.

Act on impressions to call or visit. Don't worry about what you're going to do once you call or visit. As you make contact, you'll often find out why you were impressed to make the call or visit.

Learn about abuse. You validate your friend if you take the time to learn something about her problem. Don't read to become her built-in therapist; read to show your support.

Nourish and lighten burdens, but don't try to be a Savior. Listen, love, help, and bless; but realize Jesus will save them not you. Jesus alone is the Savior, Redeemer, and the Mighty One of Israel.

Avoid counsel that is not helpful.
<u>Don't tell the person to pray and study the scriptures and she will heal.</u> The pat answer to pray and study the scriptures, sounds like you don't really care and just want the victim to solve her problem without the support of others.

Many abuse victims struggle with prayer. Prayer can

feel very threatening to her inner child and cause her to feel victimized. (See *Feeling Victimized in Prayer, p. 250; Kneeling Sabotages My Heartfelt Prayer, p. 253.*)

Studying the scriptures helps an abuse victim with problems if she knows how to apply the scriptures to her daily life. She will need help to see how the scriptures can be applied to her situation as a survivor. Your friend will do better with each of these areas as she heals. She needs understanding and empathy from you.

<u>Don't tell the victim the abuse happened a long time ago and she should put it behind her.</u> While the physical part of the abuse may have happened years ago, the emotional part of the abuse is being experienced now. The emotions were buried or suppressed at the time of the abuse so the child could function. Now the adult is stronger, the emotions are surfacing and are literally being experienced for the first time. (See *Recovering Memories through Dreams, p. 95; First-Time Flashbacks, p. 98.*)

<u>Don't say you know how she feels.</u> Even if you have been through hard times, you don't know just how she feels. Tell the person you can't imagine her pain. Tell her you are so sorry she had to go through such a thing. Tell her she didn't deserve to be hurt. Say you wish you knew how to help lift the burden better.

God's hope for His children is that we will all be part of His great work to carry His wounded and weary children to the Savior. Your loving attitude can lift a burden and lighten a load.

Conclusion:
1. Even if you don't know a lot about abuse, you can be a loving, empathetic listener.
2. Show concern for your friend by making contact

when you feel prompted to do so. Helping a friend doesn't need to be a 24-hour-a-day activity.

SHOULD I GO TO THERAPY?

What good is therapy?

If I'm uneasy about therapy, wouldn't it be better to stay away from it?

You are in charge of your healing. You decide when and how to do it. Even when you are committed to work on healing, making a decision to go to therapy is often a difficult one. There is sometimes a stigma connected with therapy. We think we should be self-sufficient with our mental health.

Fears and concerns about therapy. Many people who would go to a doctor for help with physical problems would never go to a therapist. They fear going to therapy might mean they are unstable or that something is wrong with them personally. When you have tried to make a decision about going into therapy, you might have had some of these thoughts:

- Therapy must not be right for me because I have a yucky feeling whenever I think about it.
- My problem isn't serious enough to go to therapy. It was not a big deal.
- I'm coping fine right now, the trauma is not affecting me.
- Maybe I'll go to therapy when I'm more together.
- I've coped for years, why should I change things now?

If you let feelings of discomfort control you, you will never start therapy. It *is* scary and uncomfortable. Going to therapy means purposely stepping into unknown territory and looking at your entire life through new windows with someone else. You don't know what your life will look like, so it is uncomfortable to trust someone to look at it. (See *Willingness to Heal, p. 58*.)

There are many reasons therapy is scary. Therapy may make you feel vulnerable. You fear the unknown or the pain that may result from therapy. You may be afraid you will discover your problems are your fault.

Many victims fear their problems are so deep they will be sucked into counseling and never get out. Others worry what family or friends will think. You might fear change and what that change will do to your life. You may not trust someone to help you because you have felt abandoned by authority figures. You may even fear that there is nothing wrong and you're simply too weak to deal with life.

When you go to therapy, you will often feel pain, confusion, and anxiety as the memories of the past surface. When I first started seeing a therapist, I felt constant stress and inner shaking from anxiety for over a year while my memories were returning. It was difficult to function because I needed so much energy to work through pain.

You think your past hasn't affected you until your memories become your reality. Then you struggle to cope with everyday living and trauma from the past. As you try to find healing from your pain, the painful effects of abuse often get worse before they get better. But as you receive help and struggle to work through painful issues, the future will be better and brighter than you can now comprehend.

Help in the healing process. Although going to therapy is a scary prospect, it is there you will find skilled, trained professionals who will be equipped to help you through your healing process. You can be guided through your pain by people who have dealt with similar problems and will not think you are crazy. They can teach you survival techniques and coping mechanisms that will help you progress and move toward healing.

God wants you to heal, but He expects you to do the work necessary to make healing possible. He will not hand your healing to you on a silver platter.

I promise going to therapy will be worth it and later the pain you now experience will seem as a dream. It will be left only as a memory and you will be rewarded for your daily work. You will feel peace come into your life and you will start to feel true joy.

Conclusion:

1. There are many reasons for avoiding therapy. Your fears will keep you out of therapy unless you are determined to go.

2. Going to therapy may make your life worse instead of better for a while as you deal with difficult issues.

3. Therapists are skilled professionals who understand your pain and can help you find the way to heal.

STARTING THERAPY

How can I feel safe following the commitment to go to therapy?

I'm coping okay, why should I go to therapy?

As you make the decision about whether to go to therapy, you might wonder if you really need it. After all, you've been coping with life. You're doing okay. Why should you go to therapy now?

When the Israelites were in bondage, they had existed for years in this environment. Bondage was the only life they had ever known. You have never known a life other than the one you are experiencing. You may feel more comfortable with your bondage than with the unknown. (See *Willingness to Heal, p 58*).

Analyze how well you are coping:
- Are you happy?
- Do you feel peace and joy?
- Do you know what it is like to feel loved by God just for being you?
- Do you feel your burdens are light?
- Can you understand and apply the gospel freely to receive more and more joy?
- Do you look forward to each new day?

If you cannot answer yes to these questions, you may be experiencing a brokenness that keeps you from achieving God's goal for you--to experience joy.

This section will give some suggestions to tell if therapy could be beneficial. Here are some basic signs to look to if you're considering therapy. The list is not conclusive. Once you read this list, you may think of other signs that apply to you.

Signs that therapy might be beneficial:
- When you try to listen to yourself or to others you are unable to concentrate.
- You can't concentrate when you try to read or pray.
- You jump from one activity to another and can't keep on task to accomplish goals.
- You feel unable to cope, to nurture, to gain strength from good living.
- There are days when you can't get out of bed.
- You feel nothing is enjoyable.

- You feel like you have a chemical imbalance or need a vitamin. You need something to snap you out of your limitations.
- You experience extreme changes of emotion or complete numbness.
- You continually feel guilty or inadequate.
- You feel chaos within which makes it difficult to recognize the Holy Ghost.
- You feel as though many voices or complete thought changes muffle your ability to see and feel and think clearly. You can see issues from completely different points of view. One day you have one opinion and the next day your opinion is entirely different. During short periods of time you switch back and forth and can't understand one opinion while you support the other opinion.
- You have dreams and nightmares that leave you feeling something is painfully amiss. They may seem mystical or leave you feeling as though you are in a trance and not connected to yourself.
- You have unexplained memories of someone fondling you, exposing himself, or controlling you in some way.
- You have unexplained repeated memory that leaves you feeling abandoned, helpless, betrayed, and without any capability to work through your feelings.

Although the decision to start therapy is a difficult one, if you see you have some of the signs listed in this section, seriously consider the benefits of therapy. Your life can be richer, fuller, and more meaningful once you heal. Healing through therapy offers the promise of peace and joy in your life.

Conclusion:
1. Therapy may be beneficial for improving your quality

of life even if you are coping adequately.

2. You may choose to start therapy by noticing what is missing in your life as well as what is wrong with your life.

CHOOSING A THERAPIST

How can you tell if someone is a good therapist?

What do you do if you don't like your therapist after you start therapy?

Choosing a therapist is almost as difficult a decision as deciding to go to therapy. How do you decide who to see? What are the characteristics of a good therapist? What if you start to go to a therapist and you don't like him? This section will answer these questions.

(Note: There are many wonderful female therapists. I've chosen to use "he" or "him" to designate the therapist for easier reading.)

Choosing your therapist. Not all therapists are the same. All counsel from their own experience, interpretation of their schooling, and their own values or moral code by which they live.

These were the greatest insights I found in choosing a therapist:

- Seek a therapist within your safety network. I chose therapists from my own faith because I felt their insight and values would help me to achieve the goal of healing within the safety of the truth and light of the Savior. Whether you go to a therapist of your faith or not, seek a therapist with your values. (See *The Surest Path to Healing, p. 66*.)

- Ask God for direction in seeking the best prepared therapists for your individual needs and stage of healing.

- Follow thoughts or desires that lead you to a certain agency or therapist. This is a pattern of how the Spirit answers prayers. Follow impressions promptly. Be aware of the peace of mind or emptiness of thought that may come as you follow through. Don't cancel an appointment because of anxiety or discomfort. This is the feeling of your untrusting, fearful inner child, not your adult thinking self.

Characteristics of an effective therapist. These characteristics will lead to a trusting relationship with your therapist:

- The therapist makes responses that validate you when you share your feelings or thoughts. You feel more sure. He doesn't think you're crazy. He makes you feel that what you are experiencing is real and normal for what you have or may have gone through.

- He is connected to what you are saying. You don't feel like he's talking about apples while you are talking about oranges. You don't feel misunderstood.

- You feel he cares and really listens. You feel talking is safe and you feel warmly invited to share. You feel nurtured concerning abandonment issues.

- He helps you where you are in your healing and leads you from that point to discover more of what to do about it. You feel a lot of "Ah ha! That's what's happening! This is what I can do about it!"

- He believes you can heal, you are progressing, and that you are strong for having experienced what you have.

- The past week's progress, pain and confusion are the subject of the day. The therapist can help you work on the "here and now" as well as other planned material.

    Changing therapists. Sometimes you will start with a therapist and then feel a need to change. Here is a guide to help you feel more secure to know that you can be in charge of your therapy and competent to gauge its validity and progress. Consider changing your therapist if:

- You feel you are not progressing. You receive the same assignment or advice every week. You keep working on what the therapist asks, but it is like beating a dead dog.

- The therapist decides what you need to work on and doesn't want to talk about the experiences, nightmares, flashbacks that have been going on the last couple of days. The nightmares and flashbacks are the issues your inner child is working on now. It would be practical to tap into these issues while they are surfacing to help you move forward.

- The experiences you share are met with anger, disbelief or shock by the therapist. This means the therapist is not experienced enough to handle your level of trauma.

- The therapist tells you not to tell anyone what you talk about in therapy. You are told to keep secrets from your spouse, clergy, or supportive friends.

- You feel victimized. You feel an uncomfortable threat--even if you can't explain just what it is.

- You are told to do or asked to listen to things that are against your better moral judgment or standards. For example, you are told to make out with a man (to test your boundaries) or you are told to hurt a family member for being a perpetrator or secondary perpetrator.

Carefully decide on a therapist and give therapy a try. The guidelines you have just read should help make your therapy more successful. You are not stuck if something doesn't work out. You can change therapists or stop therapy for a while. The decisions are up to you.

Conclusion:
1. Choosing the correct therapist can greatly enhance your healing. Choose a therapist with your value system.
2. A good therapist will validate your feelings and find ways to help your progress.
3. Sometimes a therapist will not fit your personality or meet your needs. Carefully look for someone new.

RETURNING TO THERAPY
I thought I was healed. Why do I need therapy again?
Am I back to square one because I'm returning to therapy?

Most survivors don't stay in therapy for long consecutive times. They go into therapy for several months to work on an issue, then their sessions stop. They continue with life until another issue surfaces and their life is filled with turmoil. Then they return to therapy to work on a different issue than the one addressed the time before.

I went to therapy for 4-6 months the first time and worked on the issue of guilt. As I talked through my feelings and did journal writing assignments, learning new ways to respond to problems, I felt I had overcome the reason for therapy. I felt good about myself and understood myself better in relation to God and others. As I felt the pain ease, I experienced some joy in life. I wanted to continue with everyday living on my own again. I felt my healing was complete. I couldn't see all that would have to be done to heal completely, thank goodness!

After a time a new issue would begin to surface or the old issue would surface again from a new perspective. Everyday life became more than I could handle. I would start to see that my struggles were directly linked to my childhood. Feeling helpless about how to find peace or fix the problems on my own, I returned to professional therapy.

March 21, 1988. I've decided to write in here after a long time. I don't know that I want to write about what has been happening or how I feel about it, but I'll try. Two weeks before our wedding I postponed everything. I cannot even begin to tell you or write what happened.

I went through an awful time. I was confused. I felt I didn't love Nick. I was frightened to death of getting married and of finalizing such a serious decision. I told my parents I did not love Nick and that I couldn't stay in the situation any longer.

After praying and crying and struggling, I finally concluded that maybe some of my problem stemmed from my childhood. I decided to return to therapy to work through sexual abuse.

I received therapy a few years ago, but I realized I had to go through it in greater depth now. It's hard to believe that things that happened so long ago influence your life so much now.

Progressing into more therapy. I thought I was

86

back to square one every time I returned to therapy. I thought
I would never be out of therapy. I wondered why I couldn't
overcome the abuse. This is how I visualized my healing
process:

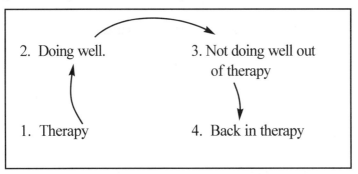

2. Doing well.   3. Not doing well out
                              of therapy

1. Therapy   4. Back in therapy

Each time I returned to therapy I felt like a failure, but
once again I would recognize the issue for which I was there.
I'd talk through the issue, work on the assignments, explore
through writing, and then I'd be back to what I thought was
progressive life.

One time after being out of therapy for six months, I
had to go back. I told a friend, "I can't believe I have to go
back. When will I ever be able to progress?"

She said something that gave me new insight, "I see you
progressing into needing therapy again. You've progressed and
so now you need to heal more so you can continue to
progress." What a revelation!

From this insight I've realized:

- All of us need to be spiritually whole to become Christlike.
- I needed more and more healing because I was trying to
  progress and the un-whole-ness from the abuse made me
  stuck.
- The "stuck time" was the time I needed to go to therapy
  to receive direction and guidance and healing so I could

progress and continue to progress outside of therapy.

I now see starting and stopping therapy like this pattern:

Out of therapy not feeling threatened by
those in authority

In therapy working on understanding
authority

Stuck

Out of therapy feeling more safe sexually

In therapy working on sexual issues

Stuck

Out of therapy feeling empowered and
supported by God

In therapy working on anger

Stuck

Out of therapy not feeling displaced guilt

In therapy working on guilt

Healing until you become whole. I have heard a comment by many that has disturbed me. It is said that some people can go through a lot of trauma and seem to survive without much help. Others seem to go through seemingly less trauma and need a lot of therapy. I don't want to say I know the answer, but let me present a strong feeling I have.

I believe the greatest determining factor in your need for therapy is the person you want to become. If you don't want to progress, if you simply want to be comfortable, or if you just want to avoid conflict, you may not need much healing because you won't be doing much progressing.

If you long to overcome, if you face conflict searching for answers and applying truths, then you will discover who you really are and whom you can become. If you go to therapy, then continue to grow when you're out of therapy, you'll become whole. Nevertheless, you may start and stop therapy several times before you heal.

Some stay stuck on one issue in therapy because they don't apply what they need to in order to progress. But there are also some who are in therapy the entire time of their healing going from one stage then progressing into another.

Most people, however, will have breaks of time to apply what they've learned in therapy on their own. During this time they accomplish many other things--growing in areas that don't directly apply to healing. Then when their growth collides with an unfinished issue of pain, they'll get stuck and need to go back to therapy for a while in order to continue to progress.

I hope your goal will be to overcome the effects of abuse completely. I hope you will find joy and peace to replace the pain and suffering of the abuse you experienced as a child. I hope you will recognize when you need to go back to therapy and not discount needing more healing because you feel you've already gone to therapy and you've done enough.

Most abuse victims will start and stop therapy several different times. If this happens to you, don't be discouraged. You are not starting over. You have progressed to a new issue. Eventually, as you continue to heal, all issues will be resolved and you will know you are healed. Keep that hope as the light at the end of the tunnel and enjoy the times without therapy by continuing to grow and learn in many other areas of your life.

Conclusion:
1. When you return to therapy, it is not a sign that you

have regressed. You have progressed enough that you can work on a new issue.

2. Going back to therapy shows you are willing to leave your comfort zone, take a risk, and move your healing forward.

3. When you are "stuck" in your progression, therapy will help you move toward healing.

STOPPING THERAPY
How will I know when I should stop therapy?
How will I know when I've finally healed?

As you are healing, you may feel that you will never get out of pain to enjoy a peaceful life. You may wonder if you will ever feel joyful. It will happen! Christ paved the way for us to heal, "Surely he hath borne our griefs, and carried our sorrows. and with his stripes we are healed" (Isaiah 53:4-5).

Ways to know when you are ready to quit therapy. If you keep working toward healing, one day you will feel whole. You will feel peace and joy in your life. The following are some suggestions to let you know when you might stop therapy:

- You feel peace in your life where you used to feel turmoil.
- You no longer need to talk, evaluate, write about, think about the problem or concern.
- You can measure your progress in therapy and you are happy about it.
- Your life becomes full with a progressive lifestyle. Going to therapy is just another thing added to the list. Therapy feels burdensome and no longer holds essential value in your life.
- You feel free from any damaging cycles.

- Therapy doesn't seem right anymore. It doesn't feel needful.

Ways to tell you are healed.
- You are able to conquer problems and achieve peaceful resolutions on your own.
- You face everyday challenges without pain, depression, anger and other issues erupting to take precedence.
- Your current problems are not connected to childhood trauma.
- Prayer, scripture study and other basic good living keeps your life in balance and makes your life happy. (Abuse issues erupt regardless of "good living" for those who still need to heal. Healing is a way to help you progress so as you strive to live the gospel you experience the blessing of peace.)
- You don't feel the need to go to therapy anymore. It seems senseless to go--what would you talk about?
- These signs remain constant for months or years. If these conditions change, you should examine the benefits of returning to therapy.

The goal is to heal completely. This means becoming spiritually whole and capable of seeing yourself and the things of God without distortions. The road is long and arduous, but it does end! Don't give up! The painful process of healing leads to peace and joy.

Conclusion
1. You will be able to tell you are ready to stop therapy by the peace you feel in your life. Therapy does not feel needful.
2. You will know you are healed when you are

handling life on your own and do not find that the problems that come into your life stem from childhood issues.

    3. There will be times you feel you are healed and you will need to return to therapy for a time.

CHAPTER THREE

SEEING MY INNER SELF MIRRORED BACK AT ME

    "When I was a child, I spake as a child, understood as a child, I thought as a child: but when I became a man, I put away childish things.

    "For now we see through a glass darkly; but then face to face: now I know in part; but then shall I know even as also I am known" (1 Corinthians 13:11-12).

    Many people who have experienced childhood trauma find they have forgotten parts of their past. They may <u>feel</u> more about their childhood than they <u>know</u>. As they look back to their childhood they may feel their past clouded like an old mirror. They may remember very little or have vague, fragmented memories. They may see only the beginning of an experience. Their childhood experiences are seen through developmental boundaries.

    Now you are an adult who thinks abstractly, you can learn to make sense of your past. You can come to conclusions from a clearer perspective because of your ability to piece things together making the complicated come to concrete understanding. The childhood limits are given endless vision because you are capable of using agency to work through the confusion.

    You will discover that the clouded information mirrored from the past can be clearly revealed from deep within your child self. With your adult strengths of comprehension, logic, and understanding, you can teach, love and nurture your inner child thus dispersing the inner confusion. Discovering how your inner self links you to your childhood will open your eyes to the key to healing.

Read this chapter to learn how to accept memories that may return in the form of dreams and flashbacks. These memories, though difficult to accept, will help piece together the broken pieces of your reality so you can learn who you are, where you have been, and why you have some of the feelings you have. Then learn how you can use your strengths as an adult to help guide and console the trauma within. You can change the child's clouded perspective to view clear, healing truths.

RECOVERING MEMORIES THROUGH DREAMS
Why do I have recurring dreams?
What do dreams have to do with recovering memories?

Because a child may not be able to emotionally deal with abuse, the memories of abuse may be buried and forgotten in the subconscious. These memories resurface at a later time, often horrifying the person who has forgotten the experience. A person whose memories are returning may feel she is going crazy when forgotten memories begin to surface in the form of dreams and nightmares.

Dreams are often a prelude to the return of some of your memories. An uneasy dream can hold symbolism of your abuse. After you have a dream you feel may mean something, write what the dream was about and the meaning you feel it could have.

Dreaming the same dream multiple times may indicate the recovery of a memory. I had nightmares just before recovering my memories. My dreams and nightmares helped me to realize there was a mystery in my past.

June 11, 1990. This morning I saw some alligators chasing after me and policemen were looking off to the side though they knew I was there. I was on a bike and started to pedal as fast as I could but my clothes got caught in the spokes and I could not drive. An alligator bit off my knee.

I awoke from this dream having a sick feeling and suddenly some of my abuse memories started to flood my mind.

Working with dreams and nightmares. Some people struggle with nightmares every time they sleep.

Nightmares are symbolic and you can learn from and process nightmares so that they can aid you in healing. There are a couple of ways to do this:

- Write down your dreams.

- Try to be aware of when you are dreaming and what you are dreaming. You are not a victim to your dreams. You can daydream about your nightmares to change the end result. You can learn to ask characters in your daydreams why they are there and they may answer you.

- Don't put boundaries on the meaning of the dream or surmise the exact details, but be aware of where the dream might be pointing. Try to prepare for the memories to return by seeking the support of friends, a spouse, or therapist. Be willing to recover your memories.

- Be willing to discuss dreams in therapy.

July 22, 1990. I'm seeing a psychologist this week. I feel odd about seeing him. Part of me feels as though I shouldn't talk about this because maybe my bizarre dreams or memories are not true, but another part of me feels they must be somewhat valid. I have no reason to conjure up such a story. I just pray something good will come out of therapy this time. I'm tired of therapy.

Returning memories will most likely cause internal trauma. When you experience physical trauma such as a car accident or an illness, other people validate the "realness." You and other people see it almost the same way. As difficult as it is, physical trauma is visual and people know how to support

96

you. They bring in meals, care for your children, sit by your bed and talk to you about the trial. People say what a strong person you are. Because healing from abuse is internal, you are not as likely to have the same support system.

Recovering memories means feeling crazy for a long while. I had a dream that seemed to symbolize what recovering memories meant to me: A *bomb drops and I scream, "What should I do? What do I do?" Start running! I'm trying to remember, if a bomb drops, do I have ten minutes before it goes off? I see fire. No, that wasn't supposed to happen! It wasn't supposed to be that way. Then the bomb goes off. All is silent. I am all alone. No one prepared me well enough. I can't remember what to do, where to go, how to get out of this. It wasn't supposed to happen this way. No one prepared me well enough.*

When forgotten memories return, they feel like a bomb hitting your soul. You feel traumatized and out of control. There is no such thing as being prepared.

You have seen a great destruction of your own child self. Your burden is great. You will need to receive strength to move forward. Faith in Christ can give you the strength you need. He can lift you up and give you peace and hope.

You have the same promise that was given to Christ's disciples. "Peace I leave with you, my peace I give unto you: not as the world giveth, give I unto you. Let not your heart be troubled, neither let it be afraid" (John 14: 27).

The most important thing to remember is dreams are wonderful tools to help you heal. They do not need to make you feel continuously victimized if you seek ways to discover the purpose or meaning of the dream. Try to process how the dream fits into issues that are emerging and are critical to your inner child. Dreams can help you identify some issues to work on healing in therapy. Dreams lead to remembering, which leads to healing.

Conclusion:
1. Dreams can point to memories you need to recover.
2. Writing down dreams for evaluation can be helpful for recovering memories and can help you discover feelings about abuse to help you heal.

FIRST-TIME FLASHBACKS
Are flashbacks healing or a dangerous road into darkness?
What are flashbacks?

Flashback is a broad term and means one of two things. First-time flashbacks give you new information that has been locked in your subconscious. Repeated flashbacks contain information you already know. You may have always known the information or it may have returned from a first-time flashback.

First-time flashbacks:
• Come in a kind of hypnotic state like daydreaming.

• Bring out information you never knew about which connects to existing memory already in your consciousness.

• Give a feeling of craziness. They are hard to accept and can give a feeling of identity loss.

• Can give a feeling of constant anxiety, great vulnerability, confusion and abandonment.

• Can be the first time of real connection with the inner child and her cry for help.

- Can put some "whys" together for an "Ah ha!" feeling. Even though you feel crazy, you start to understand why you can't think, learn, and feel. You learn why you can't function.

Effects of first-time flashbacks. Abuse victims who have repressed their abuse experience intense trauma when they start to remember their past. They feel shock much like in a catastrophe--a bombing, a war, an earthquake, a tornado. Healing from abuse can be worse than a physical catastrophe because it is internal. It is complicated to resolve.

June 13, 1990. (After several days of flashbacks) I know I can make it through this emotionally if I can learn I am not fantasizing about my abuse, but I am recalling memories that truly did happen and real feelings that I had. I just want to know I'm not stuck with a sick mind that de- sires some sexual fantasy because of an overactive mid- twenties hormone desire. If this is the case, I will exert my energy in positive ways and repent for my moral misbehav- ior and definitely re-evaluate my emotional stability.

It is just hard to believe that I would revert to childhood of all times to fantasize about sexual arousal. Wouldn't adulthood be much more enticing? I don't understand all of this.

When I started to have first time flashbacks, I con- stantly felt I was going crazy and no one was able to literally go inside of me to see things were hard in there. No one was saying, "How does she function? She's an incredible lady. She's not crazy. She could use our help to get through this." In fact, many people wondered if I <u>was</u> going crazy.

Everyday survival became difficult. I would forget to eat. I constantly said I was sorry even though I wasn't doing

99

anything offensive. I was fearful of people looking me in the eye or touching me. I would cringe at a hug and laugh in situations where I would normally cry. Those around would ask me if I was sure I was okay. I was told to relax because everything was okay. My reactions to others were not consistent with the stimuli given.

Memories can make flashbacks believable.

Flashbacks can lead to recovering memory or gaps of information you don't have but still need to heal. Don't refuse to accept more memory when you recover it because you assume you already remember everything.

It is not uncommon for adults to block out moments of adult trauma and remember them later. This often happens to adults who have been in an accident or who have witnessed a death. It is also true for adults abused as children.

A friend told me about remembering something odd from her childhood. Some children made fun of her because they thought she had a "hickie" on her neck. She checked in the restroom and was shocked to find a large bruise on her neck. She didn't know where it came from.

Years later she had a flashback of being forced to have sex with her father. Afterwards, she ran to the bathroom and threw up. Her father grabbed her by the neck with one hand, lifting her off the floor and bruising her neck. Her father told her he would kill her if she ever threw up again.

My friend believed the memory because she had always remembered the bruise on her neck and the kids teasing her at school.

What is the purpose of first-time flashbacks?

Flashbacks are calls from the inner child bringing experiences to the adult self's conscious level of feeling and understanding so she can heal. It is a way for the inner child to say, "I am here. I need your help. I'm stuck in pain." The inner child is a witness to what happened to you and what must be resolved to help you become whole. When you refuse to accept more information, you refuse to heal.

July 28, 1990. Today I've thought about my memories of abuse and it pulls together a lot of the missing pieces to my puzzle of life. I think I am starting to accept and believe the memories of my abuse.

I had first-time flashbacks at 25 years of age. I lay all alone in the Republic of China not knowing how to speak but a sentence of Mandarin or Taiwanese. I saw scenes of horror flash across my mind. I was caught up in a dream, but I was awake.

June 11, 1990. These memories are disturbing on this beautiful Monday. I've tried to be a moral girl, but my childhood memories of sexual abuse arouse me and I'm not sure what I am supposed to do with these new feelings and thoughts.

This is a lot of garbage to put in this journal. This is not a pretty part. Being sexually abused from 2-10 years of age poses some problems when cleaning out my closet of life so I can give it to the Savior to be cleansed.

I want to marry and know I cannot marry anyone no matter how valiant and noble he may be until I get through this and see sex clearly with my experiences past/present/future in their proper place. If I choose not to work through this, I know I choose to live my life alone.

God's help through flashbacks. I felt God's

presence during my flashbacks. I felt Him saying to me, "This is what happened." I saw my temple, <u>my</u> <u>life</u> desecrated. Shock? Yes! Confusion? Yes! Nobody told me it would be like this. I had no idea God worked this way. My reality was swept out from under me. All alone! I couldn't think of what to do, where to be, how to get out. It was too late now. I knew it was now out of my control. I was four months from a flight home. (See *Recovering Memories through Dreams, p. 95.*)

God never said it would be like this, not in my reality. But as I prayerfully asked for His help, I felt Him there. I had to relive the experiences and even though I struggled to feel Him, He was there to help me through. I had to heal from what happened, and to do so I had to learn a new reality.

I had to learn how to apply new information to survive. I could not rely on my past reality, I had to rely on my new present reality. I was forced to relearn who my God was, then internalize and apply truths I had superficially believed.

Emotional overload. First-time flashbacks, much like other trauma, may cause an emotional overload or numbness. You may go through a time where you have no tears, no joy, no pain. You may experience too much emotion to feel. For a long time I could not watch movies, listen to music or the news. I was numb and in too much pain. I felt an anxiety overload.

First-time flashbacks are a way of piecing a puzzle or mystery together to tell what really happened to you as a child. You can discover what was most difficult for your inner child and what your inner child is ready to work through in the healing process.

Flashbacks are given to your "here-and-now" reality to show how your "then-and-there" reality is doing. Become aware of your flashbacks and talk about them in therapy, write about them in your journal, and process their reality. This will help you heal.

Conclusion:
1. First-time flashbacks can be traumatic and make you feel you are going crazy.
2. First-time flashbacks can lead to recovering memory if there are gaps of information needed in order to heal.
3. First-time flashbacks are calls from your inner child and are a way of solving the mystery of what most troubles your inner child.
4. Talking about flashbacks in therapy will aid your healing.

REPEATED FLASHBACKS
Why do I have the same scenes flash repeatedly across my mind?
Should I try to keep flashbacks from occurring?

Repeated flashbacks are remembering a memory over and over again. They are what you think when you're not trying to think of anything. It is like re-remembering or reliving something you already know has happened, but with feelings of uneasiness, mystery, emptiness or pain. These flashbacks may come with a lot of emotion or a feeling of numbness.

Repeated flashbacks:
• Contain information you have always known or information discovered in first-time flashbacks.

Oct. 9, 1990. For days the abuse from Grandpa Gilbert has played over and over in my mind. A couple of weekends ago, I was at my Grandma Gilbert's house and she took me in the laundry room where I was abused. That room is almost exactly the same as I remember it when I was seven years old.

- Come when your mind is quiet. For example, they may come when you are driving, showering, scrubbing the floor, etc. They come to your mind when you are not thinking of anything in particular.
- Help to surface facts to bring out feelings associated with abuse so you can heal.
- Bring out unfinished business of the past that your subconscious is trying to process.
- Change as you heal. Other issues present themselves so you can continue to heal, or the flashbacks go away because there is no purpose for them anymore.

Recognizing Flashbacks. Learn how to realize when you are having a flashback so you can discover what triggered it and how it can help you to heal. A lot of times when you have a flashback, you may not be aware of it. Like a daydream, you may be disconnected from the information manifesting itself.

You can become aware of repeated flashbacks by catching your thoughts at quiet moments and asking yourself, *What am I thinking? How do I feel about what I am thinking?* In fact, becoming aware of the times you are having flashbacks is a way to help you move forward in healing. For example, if you walk into a house and have a sick, empty feeling, ask yourself, *What is causing this? What triggered this feeling? What thought came with this feeling? Where do I remember having these thoughts or feelings before?*

As you start where you are and move backwards to discover the flashback's roots, then you can move forward again. You can gain a great self awareness of patterns of thinking. You can realize your thinking links to your healing. This can help you realize the next step needed to help you continue to heal.

You may feel frustrated and crazy because you can't always control when flashbacks will come. A smell, touch, taste, specific environment can trigger them. As you connect body memories with discomfort from the past, you can be much more active in your healing process. You can process more quickly what is happening to you. This kind of self awareness will be a monumental moment for you to mark as a time you became more active in your healing.

Using your flashbacks to aid healing. Once you know what you are subconsciously thinking, move those thoughts into your conscious thinking. Talk to your therapist about the flashback; examine its purpose through journal writing. It is hard to heal what you do not realize is affecting you. (See *Journal Writing, p. 271*.)

When I was a teen, I had little flashes of memory of lying by a fence, riding on the back of a bike, sitting on a lap with a blanket over me. Because of the uneasiness that accompanied the memory, I called this weird thinking. These flashbacks were the memory I felt safe to keep within my conscious self. It was my link to my subconscious where the trauma was stored and could be unfolded later when recovering memory.

Repeated flashbacks start at the beginning of healing and continue throughout the entire process. My last flashbacks to leave were memories that came during sexuality with my husband. This made sense to me since this was the time I experienced the most triggers. The more I fought or tried to control the flashbacks from coming, the more they would flash across my mind.

I learned I had specific thinking that came with the flashbacks that kept me in pain. I would think, *I am bad if I feel. I am bad if I allow myself to have this flashback.* I had to tell myself time and time again, *This is normal behavior. It is good to have God-given responses. You've done nothing wrong.* Eventually I healed and the flashbacks stopped, leaving me free to feel the peace and joy that comes with all good experiences of life. (See *Sexuality in Marriage, p.188*)

As bad as it is to repeatedly see the evil acts of others perpetrating on you as a child, know that there is complete opposition to this. Teach your inner child God's truths about her worth. Teach her God's truths that override the evil lies of another's acts and you will heal and experience great joy in life.

Flashbacks serve an important purpose in healing. They are not to haunt you or burden you, but to heal you in every aspect you were damaged. As uncomfortable or traumatic as these flashbacks may be, they are a way of processing past memories so you can heal. Use these flashbacks to analyze and discover how you are feeling.

Conclusion:

1. Repeated flashbacks are what you already know and repeatedly see flash across your mind when you're not consciously aware of them.

2. When you repeatedly have the same flashback, you are being given a message by your subconscious.

DELVING INTO THINGS THAT DIDN'T HAPPEN
How can I discover what happened to me?
How can I make sense of flashbacks?

106

Healing from abuse is like solving a mystery or piecing together a puzzle. When memories from the past start returning, you may want to know everything that was hidden or see every piece to the puzzle. In your zeal to discover the past you may interpret your memories incorrectly and misconstrue your past.

It is important to use memories for the purpose for which they are given. When you delve into your abuse memories and force them, you can cause some events or people to come out who don't belong there.

Don't force memories. For example, imagine a flashback where you see a basement and yourself as a child of seven. You are trying to see the perpetrator. You are determined to know. Your mind is powerful, but it will not always help you remember exactly the way things happened.

You see your 2nd grade teacher. This teacher could have been the person you wanted to help you. He or she could have been the last person you saw before the abuse. He or she could also be the most safe person to put there because at seven the inner child is too full of pain to face the reality yet.

Be careful not to force. Don't make memories rigid and unmovable. Focus on healing, not on all the details of what happened. Delving means you want to know every detail and you want to force the memories.

I believe some of my flashbacks may have combined many abuse situations in one. I've had flashbacks where I'm not sure where I was or who the perpetrator was. This doesn't mean nothing happened. Something did. I have tried hard to focus on healing, not the abuse. Some of the mysteries in the flashbacks may never be resolved in this life. Quite honestly, I'm not sure if it will be that important to me in the next life either. I am in this to heal.

For example, I had a flashback of being on a bicycle

going to a wooded area outside of town. I'm on the back of a bicycle with my babysitter steering. I don't know who the babysitter was. The babysitter may or may not have had sex with a boy in the woods. They may or may not have had me participate with them. I may have only watched. The boy the babysitter had sex with may or may not have been a person who had already abused me before this experience. The point is I don't know.

Focus on feelings rather than details. What happened is far less significant than how it affects you. To me, this flashback was just another experience in the "pot of sexual abuse memories." It was not something I have worried about much, nor needed much therapy to overcome.

The experience of being taken to the woods was significant because my inner child felt vulnerable in the woods. It was important for me to overcome that vulnerability to heal. (See *Recovering Memories through Dreams, p. 95; First-Time Flashbacks, p. 98; Repeated Flashbacks, p. 103*.)

The purpose of flashbacks is for the inner child to tell her story, to call for help. Flashbacks are for your adult self to lead your inner child to healing through the Savior. Ask yourself how the inner child is doing.

If the experience is not relevant to healing, don't dwell on it. Don't dwell on every detail that may or may not have happened. The need to know all the details is a logical adult need. It is important to be validated to some degree, but not in every aspect. Just let what comes come.

Find validation of dreams and flashbacks through non-threatening research. I went back to an old barn, a neighbor's house and field. I also searched year books to help me feel secure that my new reality matched with facts. Focus on what moves you to healing.

Asking questions that move you to healing.

- How does my inner child feel about the information from the flashback?
- How does knowing this detail affect my inner child?
- How do I cope?
- What do I need from this flashback or new information to help me to heal?
- How does the flashback cause me to feel about and view my world?
- How does my inner child feel about the experience now?
- How does the flashback affect me now?

I am convinced that on judgment day if I did not remember my abuse just the way it was, I will not be held accountable for it unless I treat my flashbacks as ammunition against someone. (I have a memory someone did something to me, so I'll retaliate against them. I will hurt them because they hurt me.) (See *Feelings about the Perpetrator, p. 44.*)

Flashbacks are seeing experiences from childhood. They come out as a tool to help you become whole again. If you don't get over involved in every detail you won't get stuck and you will be able to use the memories to help you heal.

Conclusion:

1. Don't force your memories by delving into every detail.

2. Discover why the memory is important to your inner child.

3. Flashbacks and memories are tools to help you heal. Focus on healing.

DISSOCIATIVE IDENTITY DISORDER (D.I.D.)

Why do I hear voices that tell me to take contradictory courses of actions?

Why does my voice or handwriting sometimes change?

Dissociative Identity Disorder (D.I.D.) is a condition where the inner child severed from a victim's consciousness during childhood. To dissociate means to separate or become separated from association with another–to disconnect. A person with Dissociative Identity Disorder (D.I.D.) has pockets in her subconscious which have severed from her consciousness. The inner-child trauma is separated from the conscious adult self.

Some memories are so horrible and traumatic that they are blocked so the victim can survive early childhood. These experiences are held in the subconscious–sometimes for many years. This severing may only occur when trauma has been extreme or prolonged. The experiences are held in time so the child can function in the present. They come out later in life when the victim is more capable of handling the pain.

August 5, 1982. Today is my birthday and I am 18. I hurt because I'm not a little girl anymore. I want to be a little girl. Eighteen. I guess it's not as old as I think it is. I just can't believe how fast life has passed me by. I seem to have actually forgotten so much of my life. That is so sad for me.

The inner child continuum. Imagine the inner child on a continuum where you find good experiences from your childhood at one end of the continuum. You may remember smells from your home, the loving touch of a teacher, the way grandma's cooking tasted. Now as an adult the same smell or touch can transport you emotionally back to that good time and place.

At the other end of the continuum you find your bad and traumatic experiences. You can also go back in time when experiences of touch or smell is triggered. You feel the pain and panic from this experience which brings out emotions of childhood.

The earlier your childhood trauma, the greater and longer the trauma, and perhaps the more people causing the trauma, the further you go down the continuum. Your inner child identities become more and more distinct and separate from your consciousness until they become "alters" or totally separate pockets of experience. This is D.I.D. when the experiences completely sever.

Here is an example of a continuum showing the inner child. One end shows no inner child or childhood pain while the other end shows continual, overwhelming early childhood trauma. The dots represent pain. The dots outside the circle symbolize pain outside of one's consciousness. As the trauma becomes too overwhelming, the consciousness overloads and the experience severs leaving a need for first time flashbacks in order to heal.

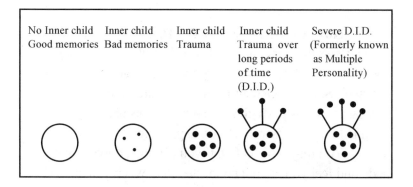

No Inner child — Good memories / Inner child — Bad memories / Inner child — Trauma / Inner child — Trauma over long periods of time (D.I.D.) / Severe D.I.D. (Formerly known as Multiple Personality)

The dots represent inner children who have been created as abuse becomes more severe. As the inner children become more pronounced, they sever from the person's consciousness. When you experience a connection from your subconscious to your conscious, you may feel like an observer watching or you may be unaware of the experience.

As you begin to heal, you may discover hidden pockets of consciousness associated with an age or an emotion. These states severed from your awareness when life was too shocking and emotionally painful for you to carry these experiences in your mind. It takes creativity, intelligence, and trauma for these states to sever. I believe D.I.D. is a gift of mercy from God to children to help them stay sane.

Apr. 24, 1994. My therapist keeps saying, "You have to listen to your inner self." I wondered what "inner self" meant. I couldn't do what I thought he wanted me to do.

Finally I knelt and prayed for help to be able to listen to my inner self--to work through the pain and allow me to feel the joy and peace I wanted so bad. Well, it came. Saturday Brian talked to me because I felt so much anxiety and he found seven-year-old Nyla talking. She feels responsible for the abuse but was charming.

How do you recognize D.I.D. (Observer)? When D.I.D. states or alters come out, you feel like you are not connected to yourself. You may feel like an audience observing yourself. Soldiers often experience this after trauma in battle. Vietnam veterans have given accounts of this phenomenon. With D.I.D. you observe what is happening.

You may have D.I.D. if you can look down at your body and feel you are not connected to it, when you are trying to deal with a situation and a feeling should be present, but a new voice is heard from within yourself or from your voice.

These feelings are disconnected from yours. You seem to stand back. You may believe you are crazy or experiencing a break down. Maybe the entire time you say within yourself, "I am acting silly. I am not really feeling this. This is not real. I'm pretending I am crazy. I am just having a hard minute. I'll pull myself together as soon as I can."

You may notice a dissociative state has come out when your voice or mannerisms change. You may start to talk in a childlike voice or use immature language. Your handwriting may even be different.

June 30, 1994. Our family moved a week ago. I can't explain what has been happening inside my heart and mind. The move was really hard on me. As soon as we started packing, I went into a dysfunctional state. I walked around in a daze wanting to feel safe and at peace. My voice went into a little girl's and I kept saying, "I just have to get up and go home." I don't understand very much about what I'm going through, but once I got here and unpacked I felt I should call Linda, (my former therapist). I'm going to see her tomorrow.

You who have D.I.D. may first become aware of an inner chaos. You have a difficult time with external noise such as children crying, music, T.V., a lot of talking at parties, commotion in a store or even in church. You may hear voices from within impressing you to buy something, to stay away from a person or place, to distrust someone. The voices may try to lead you through daily events.

To begin with, these feelings can easily be confused with the Holy Spirit. The distinct difference is D.I.D. voices exist within, crying desperately trying to alleviate pain. God's direction gently lights upon us from outside calmly providing peace to the heart and mind by which we can be strengthened. Most of the time we will want to reject truth and direction from the goodness of God because the inner child will feel it unsafe to follow its foreign and misunderstood help.

When I felt overloaded with anxiety, a voice guided me to do simple tasks. A voice showed me small steps to complete big jobs I needed to accomplish. I subconsciously named the voices when they began to erupt into my everyday life. Sometimes they told me their names and/or ages. Sometimes these alters represented basic personality traits characteristic of the developmental stage where they were stuck. They each had a distinct role and purpose.

July 17, 1994. Linda, a past therapist of mine, has told me that it appears I have symptoms of dissociative disorder. I don't understand it perfectly but from that I gather it is when trauma has been severe and the mind protects itself to allow for the person to continue to function normally. When I was a child and was sexually abused, my mind could not comprehend what was happening, so a portion of my consciousness broke off. Because the abuse continued for ten years in different circumstances, places, and by different people, my experiences caused several break-offs. They look like this:

pain "Payne"	*baby*
miserable "Misty"	*3 year old "Julie"*
protector "Susan"	*5 year old "Bug"*
12 year old "Julie"	*6 year old "Betsy Buttons"*
10 year old "Barbara"	*7 year old "Nyla"*
Woman on the Wall	*8 year old "Laura Ingalls Wilder"*

What I gather is these ages are broken off because the emotions, pain, confusion was too much for them to *process at a time and so they separated from my active consciousness <u>frozen</u> in time until I grew to an age and circumstance that would allow for healing and processing.*

Nyla--who seems to know all or most of the break-offs said there are 21 dissociations. Some that Brian and I have found are a certain age, but others are an emotion or without age. We have not found all the dissociative states that Nyla claims exist, but I do believe there are as many as she says. Even though Brian and I know these break offs exist, we do not know what to do with them. It is frightening because we could actually hinder rather than help the process of healing.

It can be disconcerting to admit that you have D.I.D. I denied it for some time, but my husband accepted this know-ledge. He had heard me talk with different voices and exhibit unfamiliar mannerisms. He believed I had D.I.D. before I did.

Entire books have been written on Dissociative Identity Disorder (D.I.D.). They describe the disorder in more detail and can give you more information.

D.I.D. (Non-observer). Sometimes personalities sever so completely, you are not conscious of the personality. You no longer observe what you are doing. A personality you don't know about may take control of your consciousness so that you lose track of periods of time. This condition was formerly called "Multiple Personality." Research has shown that D.I.D. is on a continuum and when the inner child state severs so completely that you are not aware that an inner child has taken over your consciousness, you are at the end of the continuum. This happens to those who experienced extreme trauma from a very young age and over long periods of time. Most people with multiple personalities have experienced multiple kinds of abuse over much of their childhood, usually by primary care givers.

The movie "Sybil" showed an example of this type of D.I.D. Sybil experienced extreme abuse from her mother which caused her to have personalities which completely severed. They took over parts of her life and she did not know what she had been doing during long periods of time. This is supposedly rare.

People who have this disorder work on healing in therapy so the gaps of unexplained time, or the time as a non-observer, grows shorter. Then these people are able to work to heal D.I.D experiences where they are the observer.

Inner child alters. The inner child, dissociative identity or personality is a part of you and you are a part of them. As you resolve the pain and confusion that exist in these states, these identities will eventually integrate within you and make you whole. Each alter holds a memory, emotion, a state of being. They may also hold your talents and character strengths. You can help yourself heal as you find what each one holds.

Think of D.I.D. as you would think of the ingredients needed to bake cookies. Your adult self may be the most important part--or the flour. You can survive on just flour but life becomes complete and fulfilling with all the ingredients combined into one, never to be separated as it bakes into a cookie. Integration is taking all the ingredients and inviting them to become one as they melt off the pain that separated them.

Nyla, one of my inner children, held my fun. She said I could not have fun because I had to work too hard to survive and heal. Since she has integrated, I have found incredible access to play and laughter. Integrating also means I have access to freely feel natural feelings. I feel sad when I am sad and I feel joy at the smallest sweet things. I enjoy life and seek opportunities to have fun and not simply make sure everyone else has fun.

Healing from D.I.D. Your trauma can be worked through so when you tap into your childhood experiences, you find peace and/or good memories. In my inner child memory I now find peace and understanding that is hard to express. I also have good memories of people and places of refuge.

This was not always the case. In high school I thought I'd had a good childhood. I couldn't remember many bad experiences. As I grew into my early twenties I had a mysterious feeling about my childhood. What little memory I had was disjointed and caused me to feel disconnected from myself if I thought of it too much.

I felt thinking about my childhood was the wrong thing to do. I felt sick when I focused on it. As I discovered that my problems connected to my childhood, I tried to get help for these problems and this opened up deep pain and issues. Eventually I discovered my childhood trauma and found I had D.I.D.

Not every person has D.I.D. In fact, it appears most people with abuse from non-primary care givers do not. Those that experience abuse from primary care givers do not always have D.I.D., but almost all who have experienced childhood trauma have an inner child. For a person without D.I.D., the inner child is more subtle but just as real and important to discover.

The important thing to realize is that your inner child, in whatever form it exists, is the link between you and healing. As you discover why she is there you can nurture, validate, teach and love her; you can become free of the pain she holds and become whole.

117

The inner child is a great link to your recovery. She links your past to your feelings. The voice of your inner child will often come when you don't know what to think or do. Look for her presence when you feel helpless, confused, angry, vulnerable to others, ashamed, abandoned, and unloved or unlovable.

Look for what is happening inside. Imagine if that feeling could talk, what it would say. You can uncover its purpose. You can discover this link to help you on the road to healing and recovery.

Conclusion:

1. We all have good and bad memories, but some memories are so traumatic, they were buried in childhood and must be dealt with as they resurface.

2. The more traumatic and repeated the bad experiences are, the more likely the memories will sever from consciousness.

3. Dissociative states are pockets of consciousness that were completely suppressed for a time. When these states appear, you know they are there although you may feel like an observer watching yourself.

4. Severe D.I.D. (formerly Multiple Personality) is being disconnected from the alters. You may not realize when a given state leaves and another state takes over your consciousness. You may feel you are losing gaps of time.

5. Dissociative identities can be integrated and you can heal completely.

ADULT AND INNER CHILD CONFLICT

When I evaluate my abuse, I can make sense out of it. Why can't this be good enough?
Why do I feel so broken up inside myself?

As a victim of abuse, do you often feel you are broken inside? When you try to make a rational decision, do you have emotions or voices inside of you that scream against your decision? Your adult self and inner child will have conflicts as long as you think and feel on different levels. This stems from you thinking on an adult level, but your inner child feeling on a child's level. To end this conflict, you must parent and teach your inner child.

You must discover how you truly feel, not simply how you think. This is key to healing. You need to teach the inner child about gospel principles at her level. The inner child must honestly feel emotions and work to resolve confusion with your adult self.

Understanding your internal conflict. When you tap into the pain of your abuse, you may find yourself shattered like broken glass. You may discover a child (you) at 5, 8, 10, or 15 (whatever age you were). She still feels she is shattered and is trying to find a way to piece together her brokenness. That inner child is separated from you and is there fighting to be melted and restored back whole--to keep you alive. (See *The Broken Inner Self, p. 4*.)

You learned to survive by severing your trauma or inner child experience from your daily life. It will be difficult to work with the inner child at first, because now you are going to work to connect with the inner child when earlier you had to separate to survive.

Healing now means embracing the inner child. You

119

become an ally with her and accept her developmental stage of pain. You teach and nurture her. Then she can move forward, no longer in pain, but peacefully be one with you. (See *Parenting the Inner Child, p. 123.*)

Children are innocent, submissive, and pure. However, they are not capable of seeing experiences as God sees them. The inner child's feelings may seem irrational, but they are completely honest and interpreted from the developmental level that the trauma happened.

This entry from my journal that shows some of my inner children voicing an opinion about Nick, who was my fiance. (We did not marry.) Notice how each inner voice has a different opinion. No wonder people with inner voices feel conflict!

Mar. 21, 1988. I'm loving Nick more and more every day. This experience has killed my feelings for Nick. Because of my abuse I've seen Nick as a person who will abuse and who wants to hurt me. As we've talked and I've made him a part of my therapy, my love for him and more than anything, my trust for him has grown. There are so many wonderful things about Nick.

Integrating the adult and inner child. The goal of becoming whole is to obtain childlike qualities, while functioning at an adult developmental level. By doing this, you can make decisions for the right reasons and have the ability to progress to be like the Savior. (See *Kohlberg chart, p. 11.*)

In order to truly become Christlike, you need to think abstractly like an adult, be capable of choosing for yourself, and possess the attributes of the child.

As you learn to understand and respect the inner child for her childlike qualities, you can love and nurture her at that level. As you teach and heal your inner child, she will eventually move to other developmental levels enabling her to integrate instead of being severed from you.

You choose how to respond to the pieces inside of you. You can choose how to resolve your inner child conflict. Abuse may cause you to feel unworthy, rejected, and betrayed. You may feel you are bad and deserve bad things to happen to you. Your adult self must choose how to respond to those feelings.

Viktor Frankl wrote about the unalienable right to choose, "We who lived in concentration camps can re-member the men who walked through the huts comforting others, giving away their last piece of bread. They may have been few in number but they offer sufficient proof that everything can be taken from a man but one thing: the last of the human freedoms- to choose one's attitude in any given set of circumstances, to choose one's own way" (*Man's Search for Meaning*).

You have to choose. You must decide who is going to rule your life--your inner child who is in pain, or your adult self who can think abstractly and discover answers. The more you take the initiative to use courage and follow your adult thinking abilities, the greater amount of healing you will experience. You will make good choices and reject choices derived in pain that will hurt you.

I have always minimized my decision to try to stay close to God during my healing. I realized some victims want to validate their feelings of unworthiness, some want to prove their worthiness. I made a choice--an adult decision to stay close to God. I stuck with the decision in spite of my inner child conflict. I need to be honest with myself and others and not minimize the decision.

It is hard to make yourself act on what you know is right by following internal direction from God regardless of your feelings. Through the Spirit you can gain a second witness that what you think and feel is true. Making the decision to follow the Spirit can link you to the best source of direct healing--your Creator. (See *Following the Direction of the Holy Spirit, p. 234.*)

Once I learned to love God, the decision to follow Him was, in effect, my adult self saying, "God has taught me by his Spirit and I will not deny or minimize the Spirit after I have felt it. I will follow the right." My adult self took charge of my spiritual well-being.

My inner child wanted to deny that God could love me or hear me or care about me. I felt abandoned by a supreme being, and I felt left alone after abuse and many other times throughout my childhood because God did not stop the abuse or rescue me. (See *Feeling Abandoned by God, p. 204.*)

As conflicts arose when my inner child questioned what I was doing, I had to teach and nurture my inner child. The conflicts were eventually resolved as my inner child was able to trust me by seeing the result of the decisions I made.

As you go to teach, lead, comfort, and relieve your inner child of her role, she will heal and you will see her as one to honor. You will feel gratitude to a God that allowed a way for her to be part of you.

Find your inner child. Help her heal. God will help you thrive mentally, emotionally and especially spiritually. As the Savior helps you teach your inner child, you will become one with her and ultimately find peace and joy that comes from complete healing through Christ's Atonement.

Conclusion:
1. Your adult and inner child conflict because you think one way as an adult, but your inner child is still feeling emotions at a younger developmental level.
2. To parent and heal your inner child, you must parent

her at her developmental level by teaching at that level so the inner child can progress.

3. Your adult self has to take charge and choose how to act even though this will cause conflict with the inner child.

PARENTING THE INNER CHILD

What can I do about the voices I hear inside of me?
Why do I react emotionally to some situations?

Children speak, understand, and think based upon their developmental stage. Paul wrote, "When I was a child, I spake as a child, I understood as a child, I thought as a child: but when I became a man, I put away childish things" (1 Cor. 13:11).

When you experience trauma during childhood stages, you internalize the bad experience or trauma based on that stage of development. That is why when something negative happens to you, it triggers childhood trauma and you respond irrationally. (See *The Broken Inner Self, p. 4; Dissociative Identity Disorder, p. 110.*)

Working through your inner child's feelings. There were many times as an adult I felt an illogical feeling of unworthiness. I remember trying to give my grandfather play money on my birthday. He was one of my major abusers. The money was an attempt to get permission to go on a vacation from the abuse. He rejected my attempt. I felt I could not socially live my life without my abusers' approval.

As an adult, my 5-year-old inner child, "Bug" caused me to feel unworthy when I tried to socially initiate an act I truly desired--date, pray, read the scriptures aloud, or go to church on Sunday. My 5-year-old self was trying to initiate social actions like 5-year-olds do. But because of abuse before,

123

during, or even after this stage she felt unworthy to initiate anything social. She felt wicked because of the evil acts perpetrated upon her, and those feelings held me back. (See *Erikson chart, p. 5*.)

We literally have to work through the inner child's thoughts and understanding. We do this by talking with our inner child in order to put away childish responses that are triggered by childhood feelings. This way we can behave as abstract thinking, rational understanding adults. We must learn that our feelings are not always as we experience them.

Our adult self needs and deserves to learn truth and be spiritually strengthened and fed. When we feel those inner feelings we must face them and tell our child, "You did nothing wrong. The perpetrator hurt you and you are not bad because of that. I know you are good. Children are innocent and free from the sin of others. I am going to church because I need to have the blessings and learning that come from being there. We are worthy to be there."

Learn the purpose of the inner child. Remember each part has a purpose for existing. Each has a story, an emotion, or a survival technique to work through in order to move forward. The inner child is there so you can help her heal and thus help yourself to heal. Healing means you need to go back and nurture, teach, love, and give good experiences to your inner child.

Do your best to give yourself what you need to help each part heal and integrate. Parent that part, don't just go into those parts. Learn the issues from that part and try to heal them. Don't just hang out with the 5-year-old, learn why you have this five-year-old.

Try to bring each part to your adult self so you can teach, nurture, and help it integrate. Invite the parts into your adult reality. It can be a wonderful teaching tool for your inner child to be taught and nurtured by you. Don't remain stuck, observing, as the inner child is calling for help.

If you dissociate, don't allow yourself to stay in a part you have found for too long. It is important to accept that the part exists and gratefully embrace it. Go to these dissociative parts for understanding to find why they need to exist. Why do you have each part? What experience, emotion, or unresolved issue links to this part?

Teach gospel truths to your inner child. To parent, you must recognize and internalize times to learn, then teach. I once heard a sermon on "Faith in the Lord Jesus Christ" when I was at church. The speaker said faith is believing in something before it happens. You believe something will happen, and later--after all you can do--it happens.

I had never heard this truth in the way it was taught. My mind and heart were touched by the Holy Spirit. I was enlightened, then I used this situation as a tool to parent my inner child.

I told her it may take a long time to get to know who Jesus Christ really is. We may not understand everything about the implications of Jesus' resurrection until we are resurrected and standing before God. Then we will have physical evidence of this. Now we must have faith which means we believe with all our heart. We will feel strengthened and peaceful because of what we believe.

A sample dialogue. This type of sample dialogue might occur while you are trying to teach faith in God.

Inner child: I asked God and others to make me good, to keep the abuse from happening, but it happened anyway.

Adult self: You were already good. You were not

125

abused because you were bad. God <u>could not do</u> what you asked. He can't take away someone's choices--even if they are bad choices. God would have loved to have stopped those awful acts. He would have loved to protect you.

Inner child: God isn't God if He can't help me.

Adult self: You have every reason to feel God didn't help you. It doesn't look like He helped you when you were crying for help. I am sorry you felt alone. God lives by the law of agency, but He will help us to overcome bad experiences now. I am here now. We have help now, people who care. I will help you. We will learn about God together. We will work together. I have faith God cares. I have seen it. I believe it. In time we will feel it together.

Parent yourself. Teach your child truths, give examples of experiences or principles and show sincere empathy for the beliefs behind the child's pain. Validate your inner child's feelings and help to teach so that the child self is allowed to feel the painful experiences, then mourn, learn, and ultimately heal. You may need to study good parenting skills in order to do this.

Parent yourself at 3, 5, 8, 10 or whatever age. Work so you don't allow the state to take control of your reality, but don't be angry it exists. Work hard to feel love and gratitude that it's there. These states saved you!

This is how I parented one state: I had difficulty trusting men. My inner self would warn me to keep emotional dis-tances. (I had this trust issue because we learn trust from birth to one year. When we are abused at this age, we learn to mistrust. Remember, abuse after this age will also damage our earlier abilities to trust. (See *Erikson Chart, p. 5*.)

One day at the store the bag boy shared his concern that a woman he worked with was being stalked. He said, "I am leaving now to talk to the man. I'm going to tell him I want him to leave her alone."

I told my inner child, "This is a kind man. He wants to help the woman so she won't get hurt. Isn't it good to know there are good and kind men who want to help? They care when others get hurt. I think he would have wanted to keep you from getting hurt if he could have, don't you?"

An example. Here's another example of parenting my inner child. I've included the stages of development that apply from the Erikson chart. One day in our apartment I heard the neighbors below us have a fight. I heard yelling, hitting, and cries come from below. I shook uncontrollably and felt full of pain. My inner child screamed with doubt, confusion, and shame. Pain engulfed me. I rolled into a fetal position searching for escape.

My adult self took over and I began to reason that although I was in pain, the woman in the apartment below needed help. I called 911 and reported the incident. Then my inner child was filled with mistrust. (Trust vs. mistrust stage.) She was afraid this man would find out I had reported him. She thought he would come to hurt me.

I searched for the source of my pain to find answers. I used my adult resources and began to pray for help. I imagined a safe place free from any abuse and threat. I placed my inner child in this safe environment.

When Brian, my husband, came home, I fell apart again as I shared the experience. He listened and evaluated what was being done with the neighbor. He held me and talked to my pain. He parented me with his nurturing. I felt I had made the bad things happen and I must be evil. (Autonomy vs. doubt stage.) Brian nurtured me by taking me to a children's movie to get away from an unpleasant environment and set a new mood.

When we returned home, Brian prayed for me to receive comfort and strength.

The gift of healing your inner child. Remember when you learned in school that matter cannot be created or destroyed? It merely changes. Like matter that still exists in different forms, experiences also remain in different forms. The feelings about the experience can change. You still have your experiences, but they don't affect you negatively anymore once you heal from the experience.

When you do something wrong, you repent and the experience changes. If you are hurt and then you heal--the experience changes, even sanctifies you. The pain changes to peace.

Before I had flashbacks, I had few childhood memories but I had a dark feeling whenever I tried to remember child-hood experiences. After flashbacks, the pain was all consuming. My childhood seemed engulfed in abuse. It seemed everyone had abused me all the time. I felt shame, guilt, anger, and pain at every turn as though I were back at that place and time. It was as if I was experiencing the abuse in the present.

Slowly, as I healed, those feelings eased and peace replaced them. The memories of abuse are still there, if I decide to think about them, but I don't need to because there is no reason to. The pain is no longer master of my life. I feel an incredible gratitude for the peace that exists where the pain was.

Now I remember good moments, people who influenced, taught, and nurtured me. This is my childhood that I dwell on and share with my own children. This is the gift that comes through healing the inner child.

Healing from another's act of sin gives you the ability to see truths about your own goodness with spiritual eyes. As your inner child heals or integrates, all the abilities and strengths already achieved--your strength from surviving--are yours. You are now more whole. The work you've exerted searching for knowledge moves you forward in great strides on the path back to your Heavenly Father.

Integrating the inner child. To integrate means the state is not necessary anymore. It still exists. It is a part of you, but when you go to find it, you no longer find pain and confusion. For example, where I used to find an 8-year-old lying by a fence abandoned and in pain, I now find an 8-year-old full of peace and understanding. I find a testimony of the Savior's love and Atonement.

Eventually I did not find the 8-year-old any more, just me--more whole and well rounded without the issue that existed. You must find strength to seek and find the inner child, bind her wounds, and help her find refuge and healing.

Now, when others experience pain I no longer feel engulfed in pain. I care that they are having a tough time, but I am glad I can help them. I pray for their ability to find a better situation. Being healed means feeling peace even when you empathize with another's pain.

The following is my experience with the final integration of my inner children.

April 14, 1999. I must write. I had an incredible experience with Brian last night. A friend gave me a book on mental health that talked about D.I.D. I felt dissociated from myself and this continued most of the evening. I couldn't figure out what was wrong with me. A thought kept coming that bothered me. Have I integrated?

I decided to figure out what was going on. After Brian and I put the children to bed I said, "Brian, I have to

*know if I am integrated." Brian asked if I wanted him to
see if he could talk to Nyla. I felt her surface in a smile and
say to go ahead.*

Brian asked for Nyla and she replied, "Hi!"

*Brian said later he wished he had taped our visit.
I do, too. It was beautiful.*

*Nyla said Barbara, Julie Bug, Bug, and Betsy
Buttons had all integrated into her. Jesus had held them,
talked to them, and taken care of them. Payne and Misty
had changed their names to Peace and Joy and they existed
inside of Julie Anne. They are all better. Baby was taken
by Jesus. She's all better now. The Woman on the Wall
was the Virgin Mary. She was still on Julie Anne's wall--
full of purity. Susan, Julie, and Laura Ingalls Wilder had all
integrated into one now and would soon be in Julie Anne.*

*Nyla was there to say thank you to Julie Anne from
everyone for being a friend. She said, "Everyone loves
you, Brian, and thank you."*

*Nyla also said, "Thank you, Julie Anne, for teaching
us about Jesus and for letting us be your children. Everyone got better because you loved us."*

*I told them each thank you, that they had helped
me, and they all could go away. Nyla cried tears of
happiness and sorrow for parting. She was a sweet friend
and it was a beautiful time of existing separately. She said
she was invisible, safe within the system because her role
was the fun I never had because of the abuse.*

*She also said she came out to say, "See, we told you
it was hard work." (When I learned about D.I.D., I told
my inner children that healing wasn't so hard and I
expected them to overcome. Nyla remembered I had told
them that. She told me healing was really hard and they
had told me so. They were glad I told them they could do it*

because if they'd known how hard it would be, they might not have tried. If you think you can't, then you can't.)

Nyla said, "Jesus talked to us and He told us that we were okay. He said when Julie Anne says thank you to us we could start to go away." Funny huh?

Nyla thanked me for taking care of them, teaching them and calling them my children. She said, "Thank you for being a friend. We thank Grandpa Simmons (my 'safe' grandpa) and how good he was to us. We love you, Brian."

This morning I feel a quiet within myself I have never had before. My life certainly feels like a dream. A beautiful, simply beautiful life. When I look over my childhood I see what happened, but I feel no pain, no screams for help, no numbness, no confusion, no isolation or abandonment. I feel complete peace.

So this is what it is like to integrate. Such quiet within me. Such quiet within my soul as I have never before known. I am happy, but Brian sobbed when Nyla left and I cry now. How can anyone explain how tragic, how beautiful, how marvelous and breathtaking D.I.D. is? It is God given. To see it gone--all moved into one is sad but awe provoking. I guess it may be like feeling the loss of an engagement as a wedding begins. The past will never be back, but eternity is me, all of me (them within me, they are me.) I am them.

I feel a quiet within myself. Nyla was my greatest core along with Susan and Laura Ingalls Wilder and Julie. The older three took the longest to go. I think I've healed pretty much by age and development stage. It is amazing how D.I.D. works. I'd like to learn what I've experienced. I want to shout to the world D.I.D. is a beautiful way for our great God to save His little children. What a kind, merciful God. I love the power I had to have D.I.D. I'm grateful it exists. Without it and God I would never know anything but HELL.

Do you know how beautiful this makes me? I am honored. To me each state is like a great warrior. They have each conquered an awe-provoking task. Even the angels bow to such an accomplishment. They bow not because of the warriors alone, but to Him who carried the warriors. Jesus, my sweet Brother, my precious Savior. I love you. I thank you. The world has nothing without you.

I search within myself for anything more to share, anything more to say. God bless you in your task to make whole your pain into peace. Look to God and live. Look to and apply His ways. Look to His life and conquer as He did. He did it as a Son of God. We can do it with the help of God. I know that my Redeemer lives.

As you parent your inner child and find healing, you will find that weaknesses will become strengths for you. You will become strong so you can lift another, be able to go on, enjoying the blessings of what you have built from healing.

Conclusion:
1. Many victims of abuse have an inner child who is acting on a child's level emotionally.
2. To heal, go to the inner child, or state and learn why it is there. Then teach it so it can develop.
3. As you parent your inner child, it will integrate back into you.

HOW TO HEAL THE INNER CHILD
How can I help take away my inner child's pain?
I feel fragmented. How can I become whole?

Each of us longs to be whole. We want to feel peace and serenity. To feel this way our adult self must help heal the inner child. The adult self must embrace the inner child in order for the two to heal together. The inner child exists because of your residual pain. As an adult you are now capable of resolving the painful issues that created the inner child.

Six states must come into one whole in order for healing to be complete:

1. The inner child--pain and emotion from the past stuck inside of you.

2. Spiritual help--recognizing direction from God through Christ's goodness and light.

3. Self-starting motivation--desires to do good.

4. Willingness to act--work to accomplish your desires.

5. Reasoning to learn and teach--adult reasoning or abstract thinking.

6. Awareness of beliefs--recognizing distorted thinking.

These six states are represented in the illustration below. Each state is shown as a part of the body. You can discover how each part fits together for you. Use your journal to help analyze how you are doing in each area. (See *Journal Writing, p. 271.*)

You will find that you are more aware of some areas than others. Recognize your strengths and use them to strengthen your weaknesses so all areas can work together.

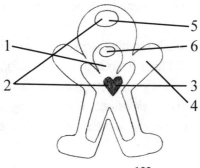

1. The inner child. This state is portrayed in the illustration as a small child inside of the adult. This represents a broken child filled with pain and confusion. The inner child is a state of feelings and reasoning originating from childhood trauma. The inner child thinks and feels at the developmental age when the trauma occurred. Her understanding is limited to thinking at that developmental age.

This area of your life comes from the past and if you experienced childhood trauma you have no choice about whether you want it, because it's there. The broken child is already within you. (See *The Broken Inner Self, p. 4*.)

2. Spiritual help. Your spiritual state is where you recognize direction from God through the Holy Ghost. This area of your life is pictured as both your head and heart because direction and spiritual insights come uniting thoughts and feelings together.

This state is your ability to recognize answers to prayers and direction given from God through the Holy Ghost. This comes from Heavenly Father. You can choose to apply basic truths of the gospel to be worthy to have the light of truth within. (See *Following the Direction of the Holy Spirit, p. 234*.)

3. Self-starting motivation. The heart in the illustration denotes your desires to do good and be the best you can be. This comes from the desire you create within yourself to grow and progress and overcome trials or obstacles in your life.

"If my people. . .shall humble themselves, and pray, and seek my face, . . .then will I hear from heaven" (2 Chron. 7:14).

This part of your life is your motivation and attitude. You are motivated to follow impressions without being forced or coerced by others. You choose whether you will give up or progress toward truth. You cultivate the desire for what you want. (See *Depression, p. 31.*)

4. Willingness to act. The hand in the illustration represents your willingness to work to accomplish your desires as well as your willingness to sacrifice and take risks by follow promptings of the Holy Ghost. This is what you are willing to <u>do</u> about the inspiration you receive. This is your willingness to act on your ideas or insights to do good even after the power of the feeling has lessened and the moment of receiving guidance from God seems gone. This is moving to do what God has asked you to do. This is not acting in order to alleviate unwanted feelings. It is working to accomplish goals because you understand more than what you feel.

This area stems from the character you build day by day. You decide to get out of your comfort zone and do. As you receive ideas and direction, you believe enough to apply it to learn of its truth. You are willing to work and risk and make decisions. (See *Willingness to Heal, p. 58.*)

5. Reasoning to learn and teach. This is the thinking you do as an adult--reasoning and abstract thinking. This is your ability to think with adult maturity. The illustration depicts adult reasoning as the adult portion of the brain. In this state you study, meditate, and ponder about your life. You use your mind to recognize when your actions are from your inner child.

This is your ability to recognize thoughts and feelings which are based on past trauma and that hold you back from accomplishing a God-given direction. This is where you work through the inner child's thoughts and actions. As you learn, you in turn gain ability to teach truths to your inner child.

This state stems from your adult self and is demonstrated through a willingness to learn and then teach. (See *Parenting the Inner Child, p. 123.*)

6. Awareness of beliefs. As you learn truth, you move to this state to begin to recognize distorted thinking. The inner child's brain symbolizes distorted thinking. When you recognize distorted thinking, you gain a conscious awareness of how your abuse experience colors the way you feel, think, and then live. You are able to connect with the inner child and see the distortion in your understanding and feelings.

You learn that the inner child feelings that continue with you keep you from acting on an adult level. You learn to recognize when you are reacting to situations using logic formed during childhood trauma. Your behavior and beliefs are linked to distortions of the world formed because of trauma in childhood. (See *Depression, p. 31.*)

You are unable to progress because trauma during the developmental stages causes feelings and thinking at that developmental level to stand still within yourself. Look at the development chart by Erik Erikson at the beginning of this book. It shows that damage done at any level can cause distortions and problems with the stages a child has already gone through as well as the stages thereafter. These distortions cause adults to believe certain behavior is appropriate or certain beliefs are true.

When you recognize distorted thinking, you realize the source of the belief comes from strong feelings caused from trauma during early developmental stages. You can then move forward to continue to teach your inner child to heal the distortions. (See *Distorted Thinking, p. 13.*)

Your body, mind, and spirit have been miraculously intertwined so they can work together to make a whole. Even though you have suffered trauma and damage, each part of yourself can help you to heal the whole. Use your strengths to help heal the weak parts of yourself. Your Father in Heaven will guide you as you learn to heal your inner child.

Conclusion:

1. To become whole you need to integrate parts of yourself that seem fragmented.

2. There are six states that need to work together for you to heal: the inner child, spiritual help, self-starting motivation, willingness to act, reasoning to learn and teach, and awareness of beliefs.

WORKING WITH THE INNER CHILD

There was a time when I felt I couldn't go on. I lay down feeling as though I could no longer move forward. My husband, Brian, asked me what was happening. I said I couldn't function. My voice sounded unusual so my husband asked, "What is your name?"

Here is a sample dialogue between my husband and two of my inner children:

I answered, "Payne."

Brian: Where are you?

Julie Anne/Payne: Lying here by the fence. I cannot move. I am so full of pain. I have no where to go, no one cares about me. No one wants to help me.

Brian: Why is your name Payne?

Julie Anne/Payne: See him there. There by the barn. He told me what to do. I did all the things he asked. Now he is mad at me. He sent me away. I am so alone. He doesn't care about me. I did what he said, but he hurt me and won't help me feel better. (I began to sob, then was silent.)

Brian: Who is this?

Julie Anne/Laura: Laura. Laura Ingalls Wilder.

Brian: Hello. How are you, Laura?

Julie Anne/Laura: I am fine.

137

Brian: You aren't in pain?

Julie Anne/Laura: No, I have good things happen to me.
My daddy is Charles Ingalls. You know, Pa.

Brian: Oh, yes, that's right.

Julie Anne/ Laura: Not much bad happens to me and
when I have troubles Pa comes and helps me and everything is
all right.

Brian: That is good. Laura, why did you come?

Julie Anne/Laura: Because Payne had to leave. She
doesn't have Pa, you know.

Brian: I see. How can we help Payne? She is so sad.

Julie Anne/Laura: She needs to go home, but she can't.

Brian: Let's take her home together, shall we? Payne,
where are you? We want to help you. (No answer.) Payne,
please let us help you. You are alone and we care about you.
Laura Ingalls Wilder, do you think you could get your Pa to
help us, too?

Julie Anne/Payne: No Pa! I don't want any Pa's
helping.

Brian: Payne, thank you for letting us find you again.
Are you still by the fence?

Julie Anne/Payne: Yes. But no Pa helping!

Brian: Okay, Payne. No Pa helping. Where by the
fence?

Julie Anne/Payne: In the bush by the fence.

Brian: Can I come near to help you out?

Julie Anne/Payne: No.

Brian: Where do you want to be so you won't hurt so
much?

Julie Anne/Payne: I can't find a place. There's no place
for me. I'm in too much pain.

Brian: What shall we do then?

Julie Anne/Payne: I want to rest. I am tired of hurting.

Brian: Can we put you in bed?

Julie Anne/Payne: I am in bed.

Brian: I'm glad you were able to move. You are a strong girl. You surely try hard to do what others want you to. You don't deserve to be lonely or hurt. I care, Payne. I am sorry you are lonely and hurt. You are very tired.

Julie Anne/Payne: I am tired.

Brian: What are you going to do now, Payne?

Julie Anne/Payne: I need to rest now.

Brian: Okay. I'll talk to you later, Payne.

Some dissociative states are very exhausting to work in. I sometimes needed to sleep after a visit with an identity.

You can work with the inner child in this way at any developmental level. If you work with the inner child yourself, you play the role my husband played and listen to your own feelings. You can respond to your feelings within with a loving dialogue similar to this one.

ADULT TRAUMA CAN ACCESS HEALING FOR THE INNER CHILD

How can I work with the inner child when I'm suffering from adult trauma right now?

What do I do with the inner child that will move me to becoming whole?

We often assume the trials of our everyday life will get in the way of our healing. We think healing must be set aside when adult life becomes difficult and challenging. This is not true. Our inner child, though broken from past trauma, can be helped to heal when she is taught about the adult self's present trauma. As strange as it seems, our present trials can be catalysts to help the inner child learn truths which will enable her to develop and become whole.

Your adult self can teach the inner child as you experience everyday trials. The inner child will be able to learn from you as you show her how your trials connect to hers. You can show her how you can face the truths of those trials. You can use your adult self and/or other trusted adults to teach truths that are currently beyond the child's ability to understand because of her developmental level. This will nurture the inner child through the painful trauma.

This can be done during first time or repeated flashbacks. The inner child can also be taught during other traumatic experiences such as death, illness or tragedy that parallel the conflicts the inner child faces. The experience may be too abstract for the inner child to understand, but her understanding can be increased as she is taught at her developmental level.

A lesson from my daughter. Here's one lesson I learned and then taught my inner children when my daughter, BreAnne, had surgery. When BreAnne was in the hospital the nurses could not find a vein for her blood work and I was asked to leave. I wanted to be there to nurture her. The nurses told me to let them be "the bad guys" and I could nurture her later. The nurses said if BreAnne saw me there while pain was being inflicted she would wonder why I let her be hurt.

Going through this experience helped me teach my inner child to realize that when she was being abused she felt the pain "the bad guys" inflicted. She only saw "the bad guys" and did not see the Savior standing back sadly watching. She could not see Him, but He was close by.

I had been asked to "stand back" with BreAnne, so I understood a little of what the Savior felt. I was able to teach my inner child her situation was like BreAnne's. I didn't want to see my daughter in pain just as the Savior had not wanted to see me in pain as a child. But He "stood back" to allow agency. I taught my inner children that just as I returned to nurture BreAnne, the Savior was waiting to nurture them after their pain.

Use pure truths to teach the inner child. It is essential that you search for pure truths through scriptures and prayer while you are working to heal. If you are someone helping a survivor, you must apply solid principles of truth to teach and nurture the inner child and increase adult understanding.

You will discover a person does not heal when the adult increases in understanding and truth. It is when the inner child internalizes the truths which are directly taught at her developmental level that the inner child is healed, thus healing the adult. The adult is healed as the adult and inner child become whole.

Because trauma causes pain to be stuck inside, you will heal when you are taught and loved with a level of intensity that combats the evil and hate that caused the trauma. Understanding of truths must surpass past pain and sink deep into the soul of the broken hearted. The love found by discovering God's truths will fill the holes of the "broken-ness" and solidify the heart to become whole again.

Nurture the inner child. Learning to visualize your inner child and learning how to communicate with her is essential to healing. You can move her to wholeness when you lovingly teach her the very purpose of her existence. This will lift her out of pain into a new world embraced by the Savior's truths and Atonement.

As you feel your inner child triggered by your adult

trials, you can follow the pain by internally visualizing where the call for help is coming from. You will be able to visualize yourself at an age when you were traumatized, confused, or angry. Then, imagine a real or created place of refuge. Set up a garden, beach, mountain, waterfall, or room. You will believe the place exists as you create the visual details in your mind.

You can also imagine a safe person who is a refuge. Set up healing baths, rocking chairs, children's books, songs of love. Imagine a person to aid in loving you back to health. Use these creations to rescue the inner child, to strengthen and love her. These experiences are very real. Take your inner child to these places or experiences and allow them to help you.

The best avenue to healing is to have help from others. It is difficult to heal alone. The adult self knows the pain, but learning truth and helping the inner child internalize truth is difficult for multiple reasons:

- Connecting with the inner child takes a high level of energy.
- Many of our feelings come from the inner child so it takes courage and faith to act on what we learn regardless of how we feel. Often this cannot be done without support because we feel intense fears.
- Some childhood trauma creates chaos so intense that it is difficult to differentiate false beliefs and limited childhood truths from real, abstract, valid truth. It takes a high level of mature adult thinking to do this.

You can learn how to teach your inner child during times of personal trauma if you speak God's nurturing truths to your inner child as the Holy Spirit whispers to confirm truth to you. With the help of others show the broken parts of yourself how to hear those words, see where they fit into her pain, and how you and God can care for her because of these truths.

Conclusion:

1. You can use present trauma to teach truths to your inner child.

2. You will probably need outside support to help your inner child develop.

RECEIVING HELP FROM OTHERS

I was alone when the abuse happened. I've learned to cope so why don't people leave me alone now?

Why don't people help? No one has ever helped me–can't they see my pain?

When you are in pain and struggling with life, you may feel like a small child who thinks the whole world can see and feel her pain. Your inner child is immersed in pain and believes it must be obvious to everyone else. Your inner child thinks adults know everything. She may wonder why people don't reach out to help you.

Why don't people reach out? You may think other people don't want to help. It might seem like family members, neighbors, and church leaders are uninterested and uncaring. Many people want to help a friend or loved one who is suffering, but they don't do it because they feel inadequate. They know very little about abuse and feel that they will not be any help. They worry they will say the wrong thing or come up lacking in some other way.

Some people do not reach out to help because they are busy with their own life and do not hear the cries for help or see the signs of pain. They are preoccupied and walk by without noticing those that need help.

Many good people want to see people out of their

suffering, but may not want to get involved personally. They act much like the men in the parable of the Good Samaritan who did not stop, "And by chance there came down a certain priest that way: and when he saw him, he passed by on the other side" (Luke 10:31). They may feel it is too much of a sacrifice of their time or emotions. They may worry that helping to carry another's burden will weigh too heavily on their shoulders.

People may not try to help you because you are coping so well on the outside that the pain and turmoil on the inside doesn't show. Many abuse victims, while experiencing intense inner turmoil, cope very well outwardly in day-to-day activities. Others think they should wait for you to bring up painful issues because they don't want to pry.

When people do reach out, try not to take offense at well-meaning people who offend. Most people have good motives for the things they do. When they are hurtful, it is not usually deliberate. At times, no one will seem to know how to say or do what you need. Know that they are trying to help you and have hope you can soon receive what will help. If there are those that want to help, pray for them that they will be blessed to be able to help you. Pray that you won't reject their efforts.

Realize not all the counsel you receive will apply to your circumstances. Most people who try to help may know very little about abuse. They may try to teach you coping skills that work in other situations but not yours.

They may try to minimize the effects of abuse or make you feel like it is your fault. They may tell you to put the abuse behind you and get on with your life. Some people will be so shocked or dismayed at hearing your experience, they may suggest you retaliate or act revengeful.

You do not need to follow the counsel of every person that gives you advice. You can teach people as well as learn from them.

Be grateful for kindnesses when they come. There may be many times you will have needs and no one will help. Be grateful for the times you do receive help. Be appreciative. Express thanks for what has been done. Expressing gratitude for what people have done will develop a closer relationship.

Pray for people to come into your life. When they do come, strive not to sabotage the friendship and push them away. Often you may want to lash out at people or to close everyone out because of your pain. When you don't allow people to help or even get close, then you can't have the relationships you desire and need.

When you close everyone out, you close out opportunities for healing. You need other people to help you heal.

Jan. 27, 1995. This morning I woke up at 4:00 a.m. to the voice of warning and pleading to wake and pray. I have struggled so much with personal prayer. I prayed and said anything that came into my heart and mind. I feel pain and confusion about who I am and who God is.

As I cried and prayed, I thought of how I need a woman to comfort me. My mind went to Sarah Johnson. (She lost her three-month-old baby recently to crib death.) I wondered, "Why Sarah?" A thought came, "Because she knows what it is like to suffer."

I am grateful to be aware of Sarah. I pray I won't overburden her. I trust God would not prompt me to go to her if it would be harmful to her.

Reach out to others and serve them. You may find you have a sixth sense for people who are in a lot of pain. Show the kind of nurturing love you desire and need. It will bless them. This is true service and some of what you give will come back to you.

Don't serve others believing they deserve it and you don't. It is important to serve out of desire, not out of obligation and burden. You will continue with unhealthy, painful feelings if you serve only out of duty.

Feb. 21, 1982. Today seems a lot better. For some reason I feel really good about myself and what my potential is. I have a lot of things I'd like to do. It's funny, but I feel on top of things. Life is good to me, and so is God. I realize that if you can give and feel and really love each other with God by your side, that's all you need.

I'm really happy about my "caring-ness" for others. I love others. I wish I could do more. I want to fill up my days with worthwhile, fulfilling things. I have the capacity to be what my Father in Heaven wants me to be.

Accepting help from others is not easy. You will have to ignore deep-seated feelings of mistrust. You may have to overcome feelings of being undeserving or misunderstood. You must teach your inner child you deserve to be nurtured and loved.

It is true that the greatest help you'll receive has to come from the nurturing within, but you do need others. You must work to bridge a gap, to allow someone to anoint your wounds with oil, to show love to your broken heart. Showing this kind of trust will help your inner child learn that there are those who are caring and you deserve their care.

Conclusion:

1. There are various reasons people don't reach out to help such as feeling inadequate or not noticing another's pain.

2. You can help others help you if you don't take offense when actions are hurtful; when you sort out advice and take what is helpful for you; when you express gratitude for kindnesses shown; and when you pray for people to come into your life.

3. When you serve others, you can give to others some of what you have been given.

NURTURING–LEARNING TO HELP YOURSELF
Why do I feel a constant need for caring?
How can I nurture my inner child?

In the scriptures you can see how the Savior treated children. He showed them love by holding, blessing and embracing them.

Adults who have experienced trauma as a child may find that they long to be nurtured. They want to be held. As they are held and nurtured, they may cry from deep within their souls expressing grief for being hurt rather than nurtured as a child.

Reasons adults don't accept or receive nurturing. During the early stages of the healing process an adult survivor may reject nurturing because she feels undeserving and unlovable. She may have too many feelings of anger and confusion about her experiences to be able to accept nurturing.

Many abuse survivors submit to sexuality believing it means nurturing. Unfortunately, sexuality is abstract. It is damaging rather than nurturing to children. When adults submit their inner children to sexuality in hopes of being nurtured, they find painful feelings of being victimized instead. (See *Sexual Boundaries, p. 180; Sexual Pleasure, p. 185; Sexuality in Marriage, p. 188.*)

As an adult, I longed to be nurtured as a child would be nurtured. It is uncommon to receive this type of care. Hopefully, most children are automatically and naturally nurtured by many people in their environment because this experience will seldom present itself to an adult.

Ways to nurture yourself and your inner child. If your inner child needs to be nurtured (and I believe all do), here are some ways to give her what she needs and deserves to heal:

- Visualize her. If you see her being victimized, visualize your adult self rescuing her. Take her away from those who are abusing her. Imagine yourself taking her to an environment where you hold her, rock her, feed her, bathe her, and sing to her.

- Tell her over and over again how you love her, how much you believe in her. Decide what she needs, then give it to her abundantly. (See *Parenting the Inner Child, p. 123; How Does God Ask Your Adult Self to View Your Inner Child? p. 217.*)

- Invite the Savior to love her. Teach your inner child what the Savior thinks of her. Teach her about His loving words to and about children, about the pure and innocent, and about those virtues she possesses. Share with her how He nurtures and loves children, how He would treat her if He were here.

- Visualize a visit from the Savior. Show your child His face, the tears for her pain, the sincere and caring mannerisms.

Show her the palms of His hands so she can see how He suffered for her. Show her His great love. (See *What Does God Think of Your Inner Child? p. 215.*)

- Care for yourself and as you do, invite your inner child to be nurtured with you. Take a hot bath, listen to uplifting music, watch good children and family movies, go on outings, eat favorite foods, and visit nurturing people. *(Note: if an activity would not be nurturing for a real child to go with you, don't assume it will be for your inner child. Whatever you expose yourself to can affect the inner child [you] in either very positive or very negative ways.)*

- In everyday living as you are busily serving–serve her. Let a smile from a friend be to her, too. Let a story to your children be for her also.

- Don't think yourself selfish when you care for your needs and wants. Think of the care you are giving to your inner child. She has to be nurtured to heal. She must learn that you love her. Then she will accept love from God and other people.

- Honestly work through feelings of anger so you do not reject your feelings about your abuse. This will help your inner child feel worthy of being nurtured.

There are many ways you can help yourself heal. You will find that as you nurture and teach your inner child you are actually nurturing yourself. Nurturing increases self esteem, eases pain, and ultimately makes an opening within your heart to heal.

Conclusion:

1. Look for ways to nurture and care for yourself. Use these nurturing times to also nurture your inner child.

2. As you nurture and help your inner child to heal, you will also be healed.

CHAPTER FOUR

TRAPPED IN SOUND-PROOF GLASS

"For among my people are found wicked men: they lay wait, as he that setteth snares; they set a trap, they catch men" (Jeremiah 5:26).

The sins of those who abuse or hurt children cause great consequences for the innocent one. It is as though the one abusing causes the child to become entrapped in the abuser's chains. The act of abuse is like ink on the hands of the abuser. It is as though he transfers ink to the child causing both to be stained. What happens to one often continues in future generations. Pain, confusion, and unresolved acts continue when the cycle is not broken.

Although you may see glimpses of what you long to be, you cannot find a way to be heard so you can gain assistance to reach that potential. Though you listen you are unable to comprehend and learn how to attain the joy, happiness, and peace you desire. It is as though no one speaks the language of your heart.

Your life seems to be restricted so you are without the ability to progress. You see where you want to be, but are unable to break out and move in that direction.

This chapter will help you discover some of what traps you. You will see how acts may have enclosed you in generations of pain with an inability to move forward. You will learn ways to break through this entrapment and find an escape.

151

INNOCENCE AND PURITY

Is it possible to ever feel clean and pure?
Was I robbed of my purity?

One of the heart-breaking results of abuse is that the victim feels robbed of innocence and purity. Your bodies may have been deprived of chastity and virtue, but this does not mean you are impure.

Innocence. There is more than one kind of innocence. One type of innocence is being like a blank sheet of paper. You are innocent when you have no experience. A second type of innocence is being free from wrong doing, being free from the guilt of a crime because no wrong was done. A child begins life with both kinds of innocence.

You have a right to innocence. As a baby you were born innocent. A young child is innocent about all aspects of the world and trusts everyone because of a lack of experience. Innocence is a gift rather than a choice. We all lose our innocence though, as we grow up and learn the world is full of opposition and much of the world is wicked.

Some people are robbed of innocence. Childhood trauma is a personal attack on innocence and is a painful way to lose it. The victim learns too early about blatant evil in the world. When you lose your innocence through abuse, you experience pain and confusion caused from the abusive experiences, but the actual memory of abuse may be hidden or numbed for years. Because the evil acts of another have damaged your soul, you may feel you are not pure. Being innocent, you won't know why you feel evil.

You may feel, "Because I am innocent, surely his anger shall turn from me. Behold, I will plead with thee, because thou sayest, I have not sinned" (Jer. 2:35).

Purity. Purity is different from innocence or being without experience. Purity is being free from evil doing. You are sinless when your adult self overcomes weakness through repentance and gospel living.

Purity comes as a choice from your daily acts. It is about what you choose to do about your experience. The fact that Jesus was beaten before he was crucified did not take away his purity, it sanctified him. Purity is what you do with what is done to you.

When I was single, I strove to be pure. I taught a lesson on morality and showed a picture of Mary, the mother of Jesus. I shared how we should strive to be pure like she was. I shook and got sick   I had little memory of my abuse at that time, but my inner feeling was I was never going to be like Mary. I had lost my chance. I was <u>born</u> much lower than her, and I was without purity.

When I found out my abuse included intercourse, I had a wrenching feeling that indeed I was unclean and the desire to be clean and pure was hopeless. I felt purity was something I could never experience.

Aug. 22, 1990. I have experienced a lot of tempta-tion the past couple of days. I've had dreams that I'm a wicked person and I've had an inner battle about who I am. Am I the person that my abusers taught me to be or am I the striving saint I've worked for ten years to become?

I spent the first ten years of my life being abused, five years of confusion and making mistakes because of it, then ten years fighting to live righteously.

I got on my knees and begged my Father to have mercy on me. I've tried so hard, so long to do what's right. I never gave up on myself and stopped trying. I begged God not to leave me now. I am so grateful God waited to return my memories until I was firm, independent of others' testimonies, and with set goals and habits in the gospel. He loves me so much, I know He loves me but He can't and shouldn't take this away from me because I have to work through this on my own. I have to grow and overcome this to be able to return to Him. And because His plan and Christ's sacrifice are all that really matter to me, there isn't any question as to whether or not I'll work with Him to get through this.

There is a great deal of pain realizing that I must face all the things I fear most about myself and the world. I've tried to hide and run from it for so long. I am realizing that I fear myself the most. I fear I'll fail. I fear I'm bad and that I'm what I was taught to be--the woman in the magazine, the woman pictured on the wall, the woman in the movie.

God has taught me to be like the virtuous women I have pictured kneeling at Christ's feet, walking with courage, seeking truth, serving others through love and compassion. Those virtuous women are also pictures in magazines and on walls. They are in the movies I choose to view.

The first ten years of my life I was not capable of choosing. The past ten years of my life I chose. I am responsible for and proud of my choices. Though I've struggled with morals, I definitely have not failed. I've grown and learned step by step and I will not throw it all out because I gain a clearer picture and realization of what someone else chose for me so many years ago.

I am what I've fought to be. I choose who I will be and I haven't given up. If I fail, at least I will know it was in the process of trying to move forward. If I fail, I will stand up and try again.

I had suffered and was robbed of innocence, yes. I felt the shame of someone else's sin, but I didn't sin. I was a child and I wasn't responsible. I trusted care givers and authority figures. They were wrong. Their acts were evil. I was betrayed. (See *Shame, p. 224.*)

Now looking back, I ache because of my inability to see the truth. I was robbed of my innocence by experience, but I was still virtuous and pure. To God I was just as pure as any righteous woman. I was childlike. God valued me and He values you.

You can be among the elect, based on what you do now as an adult. You will not be condemned and considered impure for other's acts, when as a child you did not have the ability to understand or use agency. You will be judged by the purity of your heart in your desire and striving to live like the Savior. You will feel pure as you learn truths to combat the lies felt by your inner child at the time of pain.

Teach your inner child about purity. You will never again be a blank paper without experience, but you can be free from guilt and evil doing. You must teach your inner child her value. You must teach her she was pure and blameless during abuse. (See *Parenting the Inner Child, p. 123.*)

Bad things happen to innocent people, but you can find peace through Christ's healing power. Christ can lift you up and give you hope to gain His glory.

It is natural for you to feel impure and unworthy because of your abuse. You feel the effects of someone else's sin. You also feel what your inner child is trying to process. It is essential to teach the inner child that the Father does not view her as impure.

The wicked may be without principle and past feeling,

but you and your inner child are striving to find healing by applying righteous principles and working through feelings. Your heart is the opposite of a wicked person's heart. You are not impure. You are purely seeking to continue forward in goodness regardless of the acts of others.

Conclusion:

1. All people are born pure and innocent, but they are sometimes robbed of their innocence.

2. You do not lose your purity because of someone else's sin. Purity comes from the choices you make.

3. You must parent your inner child so she will understand that abuse did not make her unclean and impure.

4. Christ has suffered all to lift us to hope.

UNRIGHTEOUS FAMILY TRADITIONS

Will I dishonor my family if I bring the family secret out in the open?

How do I honor God and not shame my family?

Sometimes we stay in bondage because we put family traditions ahead of obedience to God. We may think honoring parents means doing everything our parents want us to do to live within their traditions. Traditions can become a religion to us or our family.

When our family has unrighteous traditions, they hold the family back. Some people from dysfunctional families do not believe the gospel because of the traditions of their fathers, which are incorrect. (See *Moral Limbo, p. 10.*)

Honoring your parents means you become everything God wants you to become. God doesn't want you to pretend things are right which are not right. He doesn't want pain in your life or in your family's life. When your family is hiding the secret of sexual abuse--perhaps it has been in your family for generations--you are supporting an unrighteous tradition. (See *Multi-Generational Abuse, p. 167.*)

God doesn't want you to live a lie or to protect someone else who is living a lie. Everything you do that moves you to healing and helps you move closer to God is honoring your family and your parents. Your parents might not think this is honoring them, but God does. You have to honor God first by keeping His commandments, living His truths and applying them. Your responsibility on earth goes to God first, parents second.

Honoring parents and having a family secret are intertwined because parents carry the family traditions onto the next generation. Posterity then keeps the family secret, feeling that honors their parents. You actually honor your family when you bring the secret out in the open so the family can heal. It is Satan who wants to keep the secret in the dark.

Telling the secret is standing for truth. The family secret is temporal because we shall all stand at the judgment seat of Christ (Rom. 14:10) and everyone is going to have to face the truth anyway. If you are a part of keeping the family secret, you are a part of holding the family back. If you have the courage to break the chains of that secret, then you can help your family grow and progress.

You don't reveal the truth in vengeance or retaliation. You do it for healing. You can't be a fence sitter. You are either keeping the secret or standing for truth. Eventually family members will see your joy without the secret and may want to stand up to it, too.

The family secret is bondage. The person who has the

courage to get out of bondage will be free and able to feel joy. Family members will see what freedom is and may want to get out of bondage, too. Freedom is not necessarily physical, it can be a way of thinking. Once you have a vision of freedom, you can help others out of bondage.

Although there are possible negative consequences from trying to stop the unrighteous traditions in your own family, bringing abuse out in the open can have wonderful positive results as well. Once the secret is in the open, the family can be released from the bondage of their unrighteous family traditions. These unrighteous traditions can stop with this generation and the family can progress and be healed.

Conclusion:

1. Keeping abuse a secret does not honor your parents.

2. Do what will honor God and bring your family back to Him.

THE FAMILY SECRET

Why do families keep abuse a secret?

Why would a victim keep abuse a secret?

We read in the Old Testament that "a man's enemies are the men of his own house" (Micah 7:6). This is especially true in sexual abuse. The majority of sexual abuse cases occur in a family or extended family setting. Family members keep abuse a secret believing they must do this to preserve their family.

Each family member has different motivation for keeping abuse a secret. Each has a role to play to keep the abuse continuing and protected. Every member learns to survive by playing a role.

Families that hide abuse act much like secret societies of organized crime. They have their secret signs, and their secret words so they might distinguish those who have entered into the secret. This way families can commit whoredoms and all manner of wickedness, contrary to the laws of their country and the laws of their God.

Satan wants abuse left in darkness. Abuse is a work of darkness that binds everyone together consciously or subconsciously. Family members keep the secret because they fear the possible consequences of bringing the secret out in the open. Who is the author of fear? Who is the author of works of darkness? It is Satan.

Satan is the author of all sin. He carries on works of darkness and secret murder. He hands down the plots, oaths, covenants, and plans of awful wickedness, from generation to generation as he is able to get hold of the hearts of the children of men. It is Satan who tries to keep the secret in the dark. He tries to make us scared to bring the secret out in the open.

Sexual abuse stops spiritual progress and causes spiritual limbo. The perpetrator's secret works slay a child's spiritual ability to grow. This creates a child stuck within your adult self who is crying from the dust of your childhood. She is struggling to be freed from the bondage another's sin placed on her. As God told Cain, "voice of thy brother's blood crieth unto me from the ground" (Gen. 4:10).

If the consequences of experiencing abuse are so severe and far reaching, why don't family members rush to bring the abuse out in the open? Let's examine the dynamic role of family members to see if we can discover how each faces the fear and works of darkness within the family. Certainly the perpetrator tries to keep his acts secretive, but abuse victims and care givers may also try to keep the abuse a secret for very different reasons.

The perpetrator. Whether a care giver or not, the perpetrator has the most obvious reasons for keeping the abuse a secret. He doesn't want the knowledge of the abuse to come out in the open. He doesn't want to get in trouble with the law or his church, and he certainly doesn't want public shame and humiliation. Since he has not yet been stopped, he may believe society or the church is okaying or permitting his actions.

As a care giver, the perpetrator may feel he has the right to treat his posterity the way he chooses. In some cultures family members feel justified to inflict whatever punishment they wish upon family members. Some don't even stop at murder. There are grave consequences for this type of behavior.

The perpetrator lacks courage, willpower, or concern for others. He keeps the secret because he does not want to quit abusing. He may want to feel powerful and in control of his family members. He may want to have sexual experiences his companion does not want.

When the secret comes out, the perpetrator may either lie or make the person who told look like a liar. As he realizes possible consequences for himself, he may become suicidal.

The victim. Even the victim keeps the family secret. Most of the time a child who is abused believes she is the only one the abuser has ever abused. The child feels like the abuse was a personal attack or it was her fault.

The victim keeps the secret to survive. She believes the family will be destroyed if the secret is told. Because the child believes the abuse was her fault, she thinks she will be in trouble if she tells. This is usually the reason she ultimately tells, so she can be cleansed of the "sin" for which she believes she is responsible.

If someone other than the victim tells about the abuse, the victim may protect the perpetrator at all costs. She may feel angry at the person who tells the secret, believing this person is the enemy and has betrayed the family, showing disrespect to parents. The victim worries people will now look upon her family as evil and will shun them.

The spouse or care giver. The spouse or care giver also has reasons for keeping the secret. If the husband is the perpetrator, keeping the secret is an act of self preservation. The wife will be left to care for the children by herself if her husband is punished.

In many cases the care giver is being victimized by the spouse and so must face personal pain before helping their offspring. The care giver may want to keep things looking good, hoping that somehow this will transform into reality. He/she believes bringing the abuse out in the open will only bring shame to the family.

The care giver may actually know the abuse is happening or may discount signs saying the behavior is normal. The spouse may disregard signs of abuse thinking that believing the signs means being paranoid or judgmental. A wife may take the signs to mean that she is a bad partner. She thinks if she were more loving, her spouse wouldn't have to turn to others for sexual gratification. A wife may think the husband needs this sexual stimulation.

If a parent admits that a child is being abused, she then must face what she has not done to protect her children. Her problem is multi-faceted and appears to be a "no win" situation. She may choose to keep things "looking good" as the only survival technique that can help her. She doesn't face the problem, but keeps face in the eyes of others. She believes her own lies.

She has to in order to function while she allows the abuse to continue.

If the secret comes out in public, the care giver may assume the role of a victim acting as if she was helpless to do anything about the child being abused. She may insist she didn't know about it. Some are so upset about the secret coming out they become ill or suicidal. If the spouse had been able to respond in a healthy, reasonable way, she would have confronted the abuser years ago for the sake of the children.

People outside the family circle. Other less involved parties also keep the secret--sometimes without even knowing it. Teachers, neighbors, church leaders may inadvertently keep the secret because they don't recognize warning signs or subtle messages. They won't follow a "gut feeling" because they want concrete physical proof. They may not want to believe the victim and thus they don't act on information from the victim.

Outsiders keep the abuse a secret when they decide not to get involved. They feel helpless to get involved in a complex problem. They stand to lose respect while being put in an uncomfortable position. The possibility of helping looks grim.

Risks to telling the secret. It takes a lot of courage to bring the secret out in the open because you risk rejection and alienation from the perpetrator, family, friends, church members and leaders, and maybe even the law. There is often a lack of proof so your word is pitted against the word of the perpetrator. Your character may be questioned. Often the perpetrator is well known and well liked, so he is believable.

You may feel you are opening Pandora's Box and who knows what will fly out of the box when it is opened. For all who tell the secret, it means being at risk, being misunderstood or rejected. Each person who tells the family secret must stand alone in some way. (See *Telling the Secret, p. 163.*)

But, when the secret is told, each member of the family is given a chance to do something about the abuse. It is a chance to change, to face the truth, to get help, to heal. Every member of the family gets a chance to break the chains of bondage and pain.

You can bring the family secret out in the open as you ask the Lord to "guide me with thy counsel" (Psalms 73:24). Trust God to guide you, for He counsels in wisdom, justice, and mercy.

I promise as you seek to face the darkness with faith, the light will shine forth. You can bring your family to truth, "And ye shall know the truth, and the truth shall make you free" (John 8:32).

Conclusion:

1. The family secret is a work of darkness

2. The perpetrator's secret acts slay the spiritual progression of the abused child and create an inner child crying to the Lord.

3. Each person involved in the family secret has reasons for keeping the secret.

4. There are risks involved in bringing the secret out into the open, but there are blessings and hope that can come by revealing the truth.

TELLING THE SECRET

What will happen to other people if I tell the secret?
Will telling the secret rip my family apart?

Although you may want to bring the family secret out in the open so your family can heal, you recognize this is a risky thing to do. You may fear you will do irreparable damage to your family. Obviously, there can be negative consequences from bringing the abuse out in the open. What good can come to a family that is torn apart?

Negative consequences from "telling the secret." Be aware some of the following may result when you bring abuse out in the open.

- It can split the family apart. Family members may take sides for or against you.
- Family members may consider the problems that result to be your fault.
- You can be accused of ruining someone's life.
- Maybe no one will believe you. Your family may label you vindictive, vengeful, or even crazy.
- Realize that if you go to your perpetrator, you are not likely to get a confession or an apology. Examine your motives if you want to talk to the perpetrator about the abuse.
- Your reputation or character may be dirtied as the perpetrator tries to discredit you.
- You may be ostracized from your family.
- Your family may choose to ignore what you have told them making you feel betrayed or abandoned.

Is there value in telling the secret? Although there are many negative possibilities, you may feel that the positive will outweigh the negative. You may want to approach your family to bring the secret out in the open and start family healing.

I felt impressed I should confront the family matriarch about the multi-generational abuse in our family. I believed she knew to some extent what had happened. I felt I should take my father with me because he would be another witness to the things the Lord wanted us to learn.

After continual personal prayer for my father to feel peace to support me (and this was hard), my father accepted the challenge. He has always been inclined to support me even though it is challenging and he has not understood my reasoning. My father was concerned that this meeting would put my grand-mother in despair and lead to her death. After we prayed together, we did decide to go ahead and make the visit. Even though I didn't want to confront my Grandmother, I felt it was important to bring this secret out into the open.

As I prayed, I felt impressed that talking about the abuse with Grandma would give her the chance to gain what she desired--to have her children in the gospel. If she wanted righteous children, she could mend serious wounds in our family by seeking out those broken hearted from abuse and by supporting them in the healing process.

My grandmother responded to our visit with an attitude of self preservation. She has her own painful issues and her own healing process to go through. Although she admitted at that time I may have been abused, she has never admitted it since that meeting. She never speaks of the abuse to me or anyone else in the family.

Blessings from bringing the family secret out in the open. Even though my grandmother was not receptive to bringing the family secret out into the open, it has blessed our family in many ways:

- We learned information about multi-generation abuse in our family. Abuse is a mysterious puzzle to victims and any new pieces give courage and power to move forward. Informa-tion validates the victim is not crazy.

- My father was able to learn of others in the family who had suffered from abuse. He visited members of the family to talk about whether they had been abused by my grandfather. Each thought she had been the only one. Many said they would deny the abuse if he told anyone. Most relatives my dad talked to still keep the abuse a secret. But at least they now know they are not alone. They can talk to other members of the family who are healing and who care because they were abused, too.

- Bringing the secret out in the open gave me increased support from my immediate family which helped me to heal. They believed that I was abused and they were willing to talk with me about it. They accepted my choice to go to therapy.

- Telling the secret offered an invitation to others to heal themselves and to heal family relationships.

- With the secret in the open, the abuse can end with this generation and not go on to the next. My siblings and I, my extended family, can choose not to abuse our children; and as we heal the effects of abuse can stop.

- The family is given a chance to progress.

- A lot of questions have been answered about the dynamics of our family. This has lead to bonding and a feeling of camaraderie and caring for one for another.

- Simply talking about the abuse has been healing. It validates the reality of the abuse and gives everyone permission to remember.

We wish the abuse hadn't happened, but going through this trial has helped us recognize our family strengths. We have gone through hard stuff. We'll make it through this. We are going to be okay. We can recover, and God willing, we'll all be better because of it.

Many blessings can come to your family from telling about the abuse. You can set your family on the path to healing. Of course, negatives can also occur. Ask God to help you know how and when to approach your family. God will help you find inspired ways to interact with your family.

Conclusion:

1. Expect opposition when you bring the secret out in the open. There are likely to be both positive and negative results from sharing the secret.

2. Pray about how and when to approach your family.

MULTI-GENERATIONAL ABUSE

Why does abuse continue from generation to generation?

Why does the darkness of abuse seem too dark for light to enter in?

Perhaps because of being brought up in an abusive family and learning no other lifestyle, abuse continues from one generation into the next. The distorted thinking that stems from abuse moves to the next generation.

Multi-generational abuse is a work of darkness that binds the family together subconsciously or consciously covenanting or agreeing not to reveal the acts of the perpetrator. The family members keep the secret because they fear consequences. Families with multi-generational abuse have to keep the secret by pretending or literally blocking from their consciousness the reality that abuse is happening within the family. (See *The Family Secret, p. 158*.)

Bringing your family into the light. Imagine yourself as a person God placed in your family to bring light to the darkness within it. The Lord doesn't want abuse to stay in darkness. He wants the secret out in the open so the abuse will stop and the family can heal. I believe many people were subjected to their abusive situations because God knew they were strong enough to stop the abuse.

God told Jeremiah, "Before I formed thee in the belly I knew thee" (Jeremiah 1:4). Doesn't it stand to reason that God knew each of us and gave us assignments to do in our mortal life? Perhaps your assignment was to stop the abuse in your family.

You might be asked the same question Mordecai asked Esther when she was asked to save the Jews from destruction, "Who knoweth whether thou art come to the kingdom for such a time as this?" (Esther 4:14).

The angels in heaven hope you will face your family secret and work to overcome your abuse and help your family get out of bondage. They are cheering for you.

You can be the person that shines forth in darkness unto light. You are working to heal from abuse and you have started to see the freedom that comes from being released from bondage. By example you can teach your family about finding the freedom that comes from healing.

Helping your family come out of bondage. Moses had experienced freedom and so was better able to free his people. He was born in bondage, but was raised in freedom. Thus he was prepared to lead his people out of bondage.

Just as the Israelites sacrificed to obtain a physical freedom from bondage, families must seek to obtain an internal, peaceful freedom. This takes place within families when they break the bonds of silence and open the family to the truth of abuse.

Survivors of multi-generational abuse must boldly and lovingly stand for truth so they can bring their family back to Christ. Survivors can help their children and their extended family find the peace of spiritual freedom. Then their family can truly be one in heart and mind.

Conclusion:

1. As you experience freedom from bondage, you can help deliver family members from bondage.

2. You can bring your family back to Christ and become free from bondage.

WHAT ABOUT PERPETRATORS?

Can you be a victim and a perpetrator?
Can you be forgiven of abusing others?

This book has been written from a victim's point of view. You see a picture of the perpetrator through the victim's eyes. But many people who were abused in their childhood become perpetrators later in life. You can be a victim and a perpetrator.

Victims often act like perpetrators later in life.
When a person is abused, she must do something with what happened to her. Later in life many victims act like perpetrators as part of figuring out life after abuse. Many victims who have been abused struggle with healing because during their

development they treated someone the way they were treated. (See *Distorted Thinking, p. 13; Second Sins, p. 171.*)

If anyone feels wicked, it may be the person who was abused and now survives by abusing. It is so important for victims to face these acts and resolve what they have done to others and to themselves. A perpetrator may not be evil so much as trapped in his inability to get out of a damaging cycle. The most important element of healing for a perpetrator is to take <u>complete</u> responsibility for his actions and be willing to do what is needed to end the cycle, face the truth, and seek help. (See *Strengthening against Damaging Cycles, p. 260.*)

Ending the cycle of abuse. Abusing can be addictive. It is difficult to overcome and cannot be done without the Savior. To make a commitment to stop abusing, you might want to follow a tradition of some Native Americans. Many Native American cultures "bury the hatchet" to symbolize that a disagreement is buried and forgotten.

Similarly, you will have to symbolically bury your abusive behavior and promise you will never unearth it again. In other words, "if thy hand offend thee cut it off." Do what is necessary to deny yourself access to perpetrating again.

Once you make this commitment you can go to the Savior and ask Him to help you. The Savior can give you a new heart just as He did for king Saul. "And it was so, that when he [Saul] had turned his back to go from Samuel, God gave him a different heart" (1 Sam. 10:9). Christ can take away the desire to abuse.

Justice and mercy. Our focus must be to do what is necessary to be saved and what will meet both the laws of judgment and mercy. As adults we have grave responsibilities when we make wrong choices. Inner children are innocent, but adults must take responsibility for their acts regardless of the pain of their youth.

It is important for a perpetrator to stop inappropriate actions and realize what those acts have done to the victim. The victim must be careful about her intent to punish the perpetrator and make sure she is not hurting herself by being merciless. (See *Feelings about the Perpetrator, p. 44.*)

This book was written to guide you to heal through the Savior. You can do this by being responsible for your own actions and then teaching and showing mercy to your inner child. You can come to the Savior and experience in an empowering way a two-part appreciation of the Savior's greatest work. You can feel forgiveness as you repent for abusing. You can also heal through the Savior as He takes the suffering of your inner child.

You are not past hope. You can be cleansed and healed. The Savior can do that for you.

Conclusion:

1. Victims often act as perpetrators later in life.

2. Through the Savior you can be forgiven for perpetrating and healed from abuse you suffered.

SECOND SINS

Are my personal sins related to my abuse?

Does my abuse have anything to do with problems like overeating, alcohol or drug abuse?

Many abuse victims have difficulty with other problems in their life. They may abuse alcohol or drugs. They may struggle with sexual boundaries, with anger, or even be abusive themselves. These are secondary problems stemming from the core problem of abuse.

Building a strong foundation. Imagine you are building a house. The builder has constructed a faulty foundation. He built the house on uneven ground. You want to live in this great house, but you have concerns about it. The ceiling cracks. The house shifts because the ground is not solid.

You spend your time trying to patch the cracks and paint, but the problems reoccur. Instead of mending the secondary problems in the house, you have to go back to the foundation and make it firm.

You are the most sacred of structures. You are a temple. Paul wrote, "Know ye not that ye are the temple of God, and that the Spirit of God dwelleth in you?" (1 Cor. 3:16). Your foundation comes from your beliefs and experiences from childhood. For your temple--your adulthood--to become what you want it to be you must make the foundation solid.

You may struggle with unhealthy habits and patterns because of a weak foundation. If the foundation of your childhood is unstable, you have to go back and fix it. Once that foundation is fixed and strong, the rest of the structure will be more secure. The Lord wants you to be built on a firm foundation.

Your personal foundation is developed from birth to about 18 years of age. During the first 18 years of life, if you are raised by caregivers who teach, nurture, and guide you to do right, you are ready to be an independent adult by the end of those years .

Your foundation was formed in part by your growing up environment. Parents, family, neighbors and teachers provided traditions, discipline, nurturing and caring. They were role models or examples to you.

If you were able to receive positive experiences, and interpret the experiences as positive, you will have a good foundation to find personal progress and growth. If not, growth and progress may be difficult. Erikson shows how trauma, abuse, and neglect affects children during each stage of development. (See *Erikson Chart, p. 5*.)

Abuse is the primary problem. You might struggle with sexual boundaries, drug abuse, eating disorders, or anger. If you've gone through abuse, the abuse is the core event. Abuse is the faulty foundation--the primary problem. The other behaviors are the cracked walls and the peeling paint. They are the secondary problems that come as a result of the abuse.

Here is one journal entry from my teen years showing my continuing struggle with setting boundaries on dates.

October 3, 1981. I have had a lot of thoughtful moments in the last few days. I am very confused about a lot of things. My biggest problem is the fact I am a flirt and I don't know how to not flirt. But a bigger problem is the way guys react to my flirtations. They seem to take it as a very big pass. When I get alone with one of these young men, they seem to expect a little more out of me than I'm interested in giving. I want to be a morally clean girl. So what shall I do? I have to search in my heart to find the answer.

You can spend a lot of time repenting over and over again for these "secondary problems," but until you can go back to the original pain you will see the same patterns repeating in your life. You will think you are a failure and wonder why you aren't good enough. You will see other people progressing and wonder why they are progressing and you are not. You keep getting knocked down and can't seem to rise above your problems.

Fortify weak areas. The Lord knows that a house cannot be firm when the foundation is broken or cracked or weak. His mercy extends to us. Our responsibility is to try to fortify our weak spots as we go back to the core of ourselves to heal.

To keep their armies safe, military leaders identify weak spots and fortify these areas. If sexual activity is a weak area, tell the person you are dating that you have been abused and you need him to help you set appropriate boundaries. Then the responsibility can be shared instead of you carrying it alone. (See *Sexual Boundaries, p. 180; Fortifying Yourself with God's Armor, p. 257.*)

May 2, 1982. I think today I feel a little confused. I want to be good, but sometimes I do things and I don't realize what I've done. I express myself wrong and I make myself mad. I want to be a good, warm person, but not too warm.

I don't think I'm cautious enough with my morals. I want the guy to want to date me because he had fun and enjoyed my company and wants to get to know me better. I don't want him to come back because he thought I was desirable or sexy or anything like that.

I am doing better though. Last night I told my date some of my feelings and I think he understands. I wonder if he was just testing me. I want him to enjoy my company, but not in the way he was planning and I let him know that.

If drug abuse is a weak area. Get support from your doctor and family to help you with healthy boundaries. Stay out of places and situations where you are likely to be tempted to use drugs. If prescription drugs are a problem give yours to someone who will dispense them to you.

You need a support system. Pray to know how and

when to tell people you need help. The Lord will guide you to understand when and how to share with others. He will soften the hearts of those in whom you confide so they love and respect you instead of judging you. Even though another person may not understand what you have been through, he or she can be a support in positive ways.

When a person has been abused, her agency can be limited. As an adult you can think logically and know what you want, but often cannot act the way you think. You act the way your inner child feels about who you are, and how she sees God and the world. When you hit pain, you hit confusion. Your feelings may be so strong about something that the feelings create the thinking, rather than the logical understanding preceding the feelings. Then you act on the pain and confusion, rather than from your adult understanding. (See *Adult and Inner Child Conflict, p. 119.*)

For example, you don't want to yell at your children, but you may do it in the heat of the moment. You act out of emotion or the way you have been raised. You may yell as a way to try to gain external control because there is nothing but chaos within.

You may live with second sins. You may be immoral, steal, lie, take drugs and alcohol, or simply overeat; but you may not be choosing to do these because you are searching for happiness in evil doing. You are probably doing these things to find any road out of unexplained pain. You are choosing between an action of lesser pain to avoid a more serious act such as committing suicide, hurting someone seriously, or losing your mind in some way.

How to overcome the pain that causes the weaknesses.

- Recognize your behavior. What patterns of behavior do you exhibit that are emotional responses and not conscious decisions? When you do something that you recognize is a reaction, ponder why you act that way. Allow yourself to reflect on where this behavior is coming from. Did your mom or dad respond this way? Is your response a control mechanism?

- Feel what happened. Become emotionally connected through talking or journal writing. Analyze why you behave the way you do. What happens that triggers you to act a certain way? When you react emotionally, is it usually an attempt to gain control over your environment because you feel out of control internally?

- Resolve the confusion that erupts when you feel the pain. Your inner child reacts to pain and confusion at her developmental level. When you feel the pain, you are back with the experience at the time it happened.

Your adult logic and knowledge will help you teach your inner child or emotional self to understand the behavior and gain strength to behave the way you <u>believe</u>, not the way you <u>feel</u>. The best way to gain this insight and strength to act is through journal writing. Talking is also helpful, but lacks the complete concrete (tangible) experience to help you change from reaction to decision making. (See *Journal Writing, p. 271.*)

It may seem strange that seemingly unrelated weaknesses are connected with abuse, but the abuse is the core problem. When you parent your inner child and ease her pain, you will start to react differently to other situations and those problems will be remedied. (See *Parenting the Inner Child, p.123.*)

You are accountable for "second sins." Abuse cannot be used as an excuse for sins you are committing. To fully resolve other problems in your life you need to deal with the abuse.

Take heart, your struggle with "second sins" can be completely overcome. As you heal you will no longer need to search for a place to put the pain and thus feed unhealthy habits. You will be able to make choices more freely because you will feel a firm foundation of peace within your soul.

Conclusion:

1. The pain from abuse is at the core of many other secondary problems. As you heal from the abuse, other problems will lessen and disappear.

2. Fortify your weak areas while you are trying to heal. Enlist help from doctors, friends, and family.

3. You can overcome these secondary problems. Much of the healing will come through analyzing and working with the emotions connected with the problem.

HONESTY ISSUES

Why do I have trouble telling the truth--is it related to my abuse?

Why do I feel that what I think or do will disappear?

It may seem strange that many abuse victims struggle with honesty. Honesty does not seem connected to abuse. They are related, however; because abuse victims have been in a dishonest relationship. The perpetrator lied. He stole the victim's virtue. He broke the law, then pretended in front of others that he had never acted in such a way.

The victim has been involved in a sexual relationship

that exists part of the time and isn't supposed to exist the rest of the time. This "disappearing act" can carry over to other aspects of a victim's life.

Abuse teaches life is double. When you are abused, you learn you do something and then it disappears. Abuse happened, but you are supposed to <u>act</u> like it never happened. The perpetrator has a sexual relationship with you and the rule is the relationship disappears into thin air.

This thinking can encompass many aspects of your life. You steal something, tell a lie, or break a law and you feel it never happened. You think it disappears. There shouldn't be any consequences because the action never happened.

You may act this way, but you find there are still consequences. My consequence was feeling guilty. I felt intensely aware of my weakness to tell lies or take something, because I wanted so badly to be good and to have goodness override the pain inside of me. I set goals to be honest and to obey laws so that I could overcome this weakness. I felt so wicked because of these weaknesses. (See *Kohlberg Chart, p.11.*)

June 24, 1980. I'm fifteen years old. My life is great right now and full of happiness. My life used to be full of sorrow and terrible sadness because of the sins I committed against my friends. I lied to them hoping they would accept me better. I told them exaggerated stories that were only half true.

Finally I broke down and told all of my friends, my heart full of sorrow and of pain. I had to come to peace with myself and level with God and my friends and admit to what I had done for more than six months.

Well, my sorrow and asking for forgiveness from my friends was not enough. They all felt like they should teach me a lesson. They prank phone called me for weeks and talked about me behind my back calling me a liar and an unworthy friend. If they all would have known how much pain I suffered just telling them each privately that I was sorry and I would never ever do it again.

June 13, 1988. "Keep thy tongue from evil and thy lips from speaking guile" (Ps. 34:13). This commandment is special for me. I have always struggled with being totally honest. I showed a lack of honesty to myself and others in my relationship to Nick. I showed a lack of truthfulness to him. I was full of guile and did not tell him what was truly in my heart. On the outside I appeared as though I was an innocent victim when inside I was full of unclean lies and hypocrisy.

I struggled with honesty because I placed the per-petrator's acts of dishonesty on myself. My inner child believed I was the perpetrator--the one responsible for the abuse. Chilren internalize who they are and what is expected of them by the example of adults. I was living what I learned and interpreting what I'd been taught by perpetrators.

How do you change your thinking? There are ways to work out the false notion that your actions aren't real. You can make the past real by telling others about the abuse, by writing in a journal, and fortifying yourself as you go through healing.

I learned from an experience that taught me about consequences. I had climbed six flights of stairs that wound around a garden in an apartment building. I had my car keys in my hand and almost dropped them. It dawned on me that if I dropped the keys it would take a lot of work to recover them.

I would have to walk back down six flights of stairs. Then I would have to search through all the greenery to recover the keys.

I realized that if I didn't find the keys I'd have to walk home, break into my apartment and get another set of keys. I'd have to walk back and get my car later. The consequences weren't small even though the act of dropping the keys seemed small--an easy quick act.

If I had actually dropped the keys, I would have had to find them before I could go home. I couldn't pretend it didn't happen. This experience helped me make an association between my childhood experience and the consequences of acting honestly. (See *Second Sins, p. 171.*)

The way we act is real and must be resolved before we can go home to our Heavenly Father. We will need to work through our thinking about honesty. When we understand why we think the way we do, we will be able to change our actions. As we work to accomplish this through healing and repentance, we will gain keys necessary to return to our Heavenly Father.

Conclusion:

1. A victim's problems with dishonesty often stem from the dishonesty in her abuse relationships.

2. Because the abuse relationship seemed to disappear, the victim may think other consequences will disappear as well.

SEXUAL BOUNDARIES

I want to have strict sexual boundaries, so why do I struggle with sexuality in every relationship?

Why do I feel trapped every time I get in a serious relationship?

Many people who have experienced abuse have issues with sexual boundaries. Some become promiscuous while others sicken at the thought of any physical intimacy at all. Some abuse victims refuse to be involved with the opposite sex. Others may even turn to their own sex for physical companionship and have sexual relationships. Some victims have many relationships at once, controlling and manipulating, then feeling helplessly victimized and out of control.

Sexual abuse gives a distorted view of sexuality. This may mean that you struggle with sexuality in adult years, long after the abuse is over. In your marriage or dating experiences you may feel you don't have personal boundaries. (See *How Do I Strengthen Myself?* p. 265.)

Parallels between relationships and abuse.
Relationships with the opposite sex often put you in the same environment as you were in during abuse. You are alone with another person and you wonder about your partner's expectations. If your companion wants to kiss you, you may feel you have no right to refuse. Kissing may make you feel like a victim.

I couldn't seem to keep a relationship in balance. I felt like I was in charge of a big dam. I was responsible to make sure no water came on my side of the wall. My date was on the other side of the dam. I wanted to let him come over, but the water would always start to seep through with him. If he kissed me, it was like a hole was made in the wall and I imagined that if I allowed him to stay, the hole would become bigger and the dam would break. I would be destroyed-- engulfed in the water.

Many abuse survivors want to feel safe in sexual situations, but they are unable to act the way they desire. They feel they have no control over the physical part of a relationship, that they must succumb to anything a man wants. Any type of physical relationship may cause the victim to relive her feelings of abuse over and over again.

You may feel trapped in any relationship that becomes at all physical. You learned to accommodate your abusers and so you automatically respond to relationships as though you are with a perpetrator. You were trained to please selfish people, now it still may be hard to say no to someone who is in a relationship to satisfy his own desires.

I responded the way I had been trained by my abusers rather than the way I believed was healthy. Most of my memories of abuse were buried and hidden, but I felt paralyzed to respond morally like I wanted to.

I wanted to be moral and knew it was right to be morally clean. I knew I should be a virtuous woman "for her price is far above rubies" (Prov. 31:10). All the sermons about sexuality made me feel worthless and hypocritical. I thought I destroyed everything good because of my inability to apply moral principles.

I felt responsible to be completely in charge of sexuality by myself. I was to keep it in control. I needed affection, so dates would misinterpret this as wanting a kiss. I knew no boundaries between this and sexual behavior.

There was a distinct difference to me between sexuality and affection, but in relations, affection advanced quickly to sexuality. I felt I had no rights to my own body. Sexuality was being trapped in the hell I knew from my childhood abuse.

Techniques to stay sexually clean. Many victims feel helpless to fix this dilemma, so they try survival techniques to help stay sexually clean. Here are a few:

Control the relationship. Many victims use sex as a

control. If they are pressured to have a sexual relationship or if they feel their partner does not want to have a sexual relationship, they may test the commitment to be in control.

When she marries, a woman who uses control as her coping mechanism will try to stop a sexual relationship from happening or will attempt to regulate the amount of sex in the relationship. When you get married, you are "trapped" in a sexual relationship, in other words you wait for sex to happen. A man's sexual needs are usually stronger than a woman's and sexuality seems inevitable in a relationship.

For the woman who has experienced abuse, the sexual act repeats the abuse. In marriage, sex parallels abuse in that it is inevitable and you feel it is on the verge of happening at any time. You feel your one boundary is to control when or if sex will happen. (See *Sexuality in Marriage, p. 188.*)

It is dangerous for an abuse victim to think she can control her physical relationship if she struggles with boundaries. In dating, she may be better off ending the relationship until she heals enough to have personal boundaries.

Create fantasy relationships. Sometimes the only safe relationship is a fantasy relationship. Relationships may be a fantasy because you imagine something that isn't there. The person lives far away so you don't see him much or you imagine yourself in a relationship that doesn't exist. Sometimes you are in a real relationship but you make it a fantasy giving the person attributes they don't possess. Fantasy relationships give a feeling of safety.

I experienced a ten-year fantasy relationship. Because we lived in different cities and didn't see each other frequently, I could fantasize and reconcile anything I didn't like because we were apart a lot.

This young man came from a different lifestyle than I did

which made him seem safe. He was raised differently (religiously, socio-economically, educationally). We were different in just about every area. I wanted what he had, but I felt unworthy to deserve his lifestyle. His whole lifestyle was a wonderful fantasy to me.

While I was a nanny in Hawaii, I wrote to a friend at home. This was also a fantasy relationship. I could imagine a serious relationship because he was far away. The distance gave me a feeling of safety. When we got together, fantasy turned to reality. I realized we had very little in common. The relationship only worked when we were apart.

Destroy the relationship. You may find your only coping device is to destroy a relationship when it becomes physical. You might not have the ability to say no when someone asks you out. You, like many abuse victims, may have no physical boundaries while you are on a date.

When I was single, I would pray about what to do in these relationships. Over and over again I felt guided to break off relationships. The only option I felt I had was to destroy relationships in order to stay sexually clean.

There are many ways to destroy a relationship. The most obvious is that you break off the relationship and quit seeing each other. But destroying a relationship can be done very subtly too. You may not even realize you are destroying relationships. You might be very critical of the other person, thus justifying a reason for the break up. You might make yourself unavailable so the relationship is hard to maintain.

You might even make yourself hard to like, testing whether the other person will still accept you as you act in unloving and unlovable ways. Some women test the other person by making themselves look and act unattractive.

You may even destroy friendships with young men

because you don't realize relationships swing on a pendulum. You think you must either be in a friendship or a dating relationship. You cannot be in both.

Looking back, I realize I couldn't have a healthy relationship until I healed. My boundaries had been destroyed and my ability to sustain a healthy relationship without knowing about the abuse was almost impossible. I needed to heal the fears and perceptions of my inner child in order to be safe with someone.

These three coping strategies may help you with sexual boundaries, but they will not lead to healthy, long-term relationships. In order to establish and maintain a healthy relationship, you will need to utilize appropriate strategies as a way of giving yourself some power and control. As you begin to heal, you will be able to trust again. You will be able to trust yourself and trust others which will lead to healthy and long-term relationships.

Conclusion:

1. Many abuse victims struggle with sexual boundaries.

2. To give themselves boundaries, many abuse victims destroy relationships, create fantasy relationships, or manipulate or control relationships.

SEXUAL PLEASURE

Was I sinful because I felt physical pleasure during abuse?

Because I felt pleasure, does this mean I wanted to be abused and was a willing participant?

When we think of the feelings connected with sexual abuse, we usually think of pain and trauma. It is confusing to consider that an abuse victim may also feel pleasure. Feelings of pleasure may cause her to wonder if she wanted the abuse and was a willing participant.

During my healing process I heard very few people talk about pleasure. I only heard about pain. This was a problem for me because during flashbacks I felt a tremendous amount of physical pleasure from my childhood abuse. This made dealing with flashbacks so confusing.

I was abused for years but I had little memory of physical pain from the abuse; my body felt an enormous amount of pleasure. This caused me to believe that I must have been guilty in the abuse because I felt I was a full participant in the sexual experience.

How do you interpret feelings of pleasure? I felt my body had betrayed me because of the intense pleasure I felt from repeated sexual stimulation. I felt responsible for the act as though I was the one knowingly choosing wrong. I believed I must have been evil as a child or as an adult to feel pleasure at the memory of abuse. If my experience was abusive, it should have been physically painful.

This is not how God sees it. You were childlike. Your body was responding to sexual stimulation the way God created it to respond. There is nothing evil about this. Sexual feelings are good, but are meant for the time and situations God has commanded which is within marriage as an adult. Your perpetrator broke God's commandments, your child self responded honestly to how God created your body.

The adult or older person who chose to have sexual experience outside of this commanded plan was acting against the will of God. His act was sinful. Your response was honest. I feel strongly this is how God feels. Recognizing this has helped me to work through this issue in my own healing.

God created our body to feel pleasure. It was not easy for me to get over my misunderstanding about pleasure. But through the Holy Spirit I learned that God created my body to feel pleasure and if someone stimulated my body enough, even as a baby I would feel pleasure. The perpetrator's goal was to cause me to feel pleasure and this was partly why he abused. He wanted to have control and if I felt pleasure, he was in control.

As an adult I can control my bodily responses and not feel pleasure when I choose not to. As a child I was without these protective devices. I didn't know how to guard myself. I was without experience.

I totally trusted, and my soul--body and spirit-- responded honestly to anything that happened to it. When I was sad, I wept. When I was happy I laughed with great joy. When I was scared, I cried out in fear. I was completely honest with myself and others then.

As adults we learn to camouflage what we feel. We may laugh when we feel pain. We may be angry when we feel scared. We may feel numb at a sexual touch. These are learned devices to protect ourselves from being vulnerable to others.

When the Savior said to become as a little child he may have been saying, "Open yourself to me. Be honest with your feelings, thoughts, and intents. Shed your protective devices and let things be as they really are. Come before me, pure and without guile, and I will heal you." This is being pure before him. This is being honest in how you think and feel, being without pretense or walls. It is just letting out what is inside the way a child would.

It can be disconcerting to feel pleasure in connection with abuse. You must realize that your body reacted to physical stimulation in the way it was created. Responding differently, pretending or forcing yourself to respond differently than what is natural, is called guile. As a child you were without guile.

As an adult you can be pure and without guile. The scriptures say, "Blessed is the man unto whom the Lord imputeth not iniquity, and in whose spirit there is no guile" (Ps. 32:2). When you become like a child you are freed to accept and be grateful for how your body responds and is created. You will not feel you were evil because as a child you honestly responded to a sexual touch.

Conclusion:

1. You may feel pleasure, rather than pain when you are abused.

2. Feelings of pleasure may make you feel evil or betrayed by your body.

3. Your body was made to feel pleasure. A child feels honestly and without pretense.

SEXUALITY IN MARRIAGE

How can I ever let someone touch me again?
How can I let my husband know how I feel about sexual relations?

Sexuality is one of the most difficult issues to resolve when healing from abuse. If the abuse was sexual, you may have confused and negative feelings about sexual relationships which extend to adulthood. Even when you experience sexual relations within the sacred bonds of marriage with a husband who "loveth his wife" (Eph. 5:28) and "nourisheth and cherisheth" (v. 29) her, you may feel you are reliving the abuse of your childhood.

For years I associated sexuality with abuse, mental

confusion, and emotional pain. I could never be close to my husband without feeling victimized and trapped, praying for sexual relations to be over. My adult self saw that my husband was kind and trying hard to be ever so loving, but sexual relations were still very difficult.

My husband wasn't the problem, even though I wanted sexuality to be his problem because I felt helpless to change. Of course the pain came from my inner child. I had been incapable of controlling the painful situation as a child and my inner child was wounded. As an adult I developed some coping strategies to help me heal. These may be helpful for you.

Don't pretend you are okay. When I was little, I pretended in order to survive. I had to. My marriage, however, was not a relationship based on selfishness. I had to have the courage to be honest. My husband and I started to talk about potential problems before we were even married. I wrote some concerns in my journal:

August 12, 1990. I am writing some homework assigned by my therapist. I'm to write a letter to Brian telling him the things he'll need to know about me and my expectations as a husband before I marry him.

Dear Brian, In our relationship I want your goals and my goals to become our goals. I feel these are important. People say that sex in a marriage takes little time compared to all the living together and working through problems, etc. But it is also what keeps the marriage bond together and unique from other relationships.

I need my partner to see sex from reverent eyes. I don't want our personal relationship made light of. I need to marry a man who will help me see sex as a sacred act

God designed to create life and to bond our marriage.

When I make love to my husband I never want to feel like I am less virtuous a person after than I was before. I want to learn that I can be beautiful, virtuous, and praiseworthy. Even as I am physically making love, if I feel I am a slut or a prostitute or an object just to satisfy a man's desires I will not stay in that marriage.

I cannot be a split person, one who is beautiful and virtuous during the day and a seductive sexy woman in a teddy at night. I want my sexual relationship with my husband to go hand in hand with our beliefs in the gospel and for our relationship to be treated with sacred respect. I don't know how to do this and I fear more than anything that I will never master this in a marriage. I can't marry and keep a good, happy marriage without us learning this principle.

Communication continued after we were married. I had to be honest when we were intimate. This was hard on my husband at times, but it was powerful in helping me heal. My husband loved <u>me</u>. He did not want me to pretend I was okay when I wasn't. He wanted to protect and care for me, not make me feel victimized.

Mar. 28, 1993. Brian is patient when I don't want a relationship and he accepts when I do. But he does not try to romantically increase my love and feelings. This is the major problem for me. I resent him having sexual fulfillment and me nothing. I resent feeling I don't deserve things like romance, going to the beach, or a night out.

If I'd stop feeling so guilty for needing or wanting anything, maybe I'd be able to help him. (At this point I only feel angry and just think I should keep still until I feel better.)

I don't know what to do about it, but I do feel that after years of build up, it won't just go away. I'll have to work through it. Now is not the time to give up.

Don't fight pleasurable flash backs. I learned through prayer and the scriptures that God created our bodies as a gift and our body should feel pleasure. The fact I felt pleasure during abuse showed how God had created my body to feel.

Instead of fighting flashbacks of pleasure, I would remind myself this is how God created my body. I was okay. What my abusers did was <u>not</u> okay. My feelings were normal. There would be something wrong with my body if it did not know how to feel pleasure.

Apr. 19, 1991. Yesterday I was half asleep and half awake when I had some flashbacks about my childhood abuse. The negative thoughts and feelings of the abuse left, then I saw Brian and I getting married. I could see Brian clearly and I felt at peace being married to him.

I saw us together sexually and learned that sexuality is good. I felt many of the same physical sensations as I had during the abuse. But spiritually I was full of peace and light. I heard the words "Julie, this is how moral you would be. This is Brian, this is good. This isn't just anyone, this is Brian and it is right."

It was so amazing because it felt so opposite, yet the same as the abuse. It felt natural and good and peaceful. I thought, I don't completely understand why this was so different. Then a thought came to me that the difference between sexuality in marriage and sexual abuse was like the difference between a person committing suicide or dying of old age. The first experience would be terrifying, unnatural, and wrong. The second experience would be peaceful, natural, and very good. Both experiences bring death, but one is of God and the other is of Satan.

Pray with your husband about your sexual relationship. In the beginning this was almost impossible for me to do because I thought we should not do this. I thought it was wrong to ask for help with sexuality and I didn't even know what to say.

My husband led in prayer soliciting help on how we could become closer to one another through sexuality. Hearing his sincere, humble prayers helped me to realize that God really does care about sexuality in our marriages. He wants us to be one, to love physically as well as emotionally. I learned I could and should pray believing God would answer.

Satan strives to stop good sexual relationships and start unhealthy damaging ones. God wants couples to experience sexuality in the sacred light for which it is meant. When we pray for help on how to have a better relationship, the influence of the adversary will be lessened.

Choose to work on sexuality. When the pain is new, when you're just starting a new phase of healing, when you are feeling a lot of trauma already, this is not the time to expect sexuality to be different from the abuse. Do not have unrealistic expectations that sexual problems will be resolved quickly.

Sexual abuse causes a complex problem with sexuality. Layers of pain must peel away. Learning the complexity of emotions and sacredness of sexuality will not be easy The pain must come out before joy and pleasure can be felt.

June 10, 1993. Brian and I have been going to visit

192

Howard North (a psychologist) to receive help concerning our intimate relationship. I have struggled to feel and accept love both physically and emotionally since I've worked on my abuse. I guess the major problem has been my fear to trust, my need to control, and the emotional pain of accepting affectionate, tender love.

The whole act of love between a husband and a wife is so difficult, complex and hard for me to sort out. Since I've been seeing Howard North, I wonder if I'm going forward or back. I have a lot to learn. Some days I feel like giving up, but I know that if I sacrifice a little and keep pressing forward, God will not let me down.

There were many times I chose to have a sexual relationship with my husband knowing it would be hard, knowing I would feel emotional turmoil. But to avoid a sexual relationship with my spouse was to avoid working through the pain.

I knew my husband loved me and even though he played what was a confusing role to my inner child--almost a perpetrator--he was also my loving partner. At first I silently cried alone not wanting him to know my pain. Many times later he held me as I cried, as I spilled out pain and confusion about the many different issues which erupted from sexual contact. This was good because as the pain lessened, my husband has changed from a threat to my inner child—one who would subject me to pain--to a hero who has helped me work through the painful acts of others and taught me how to accept and want to give love.

Don't feel forced to work on sexuality, but do this when you choose to. I now look at my willingness to honestly work on my sexuality as work on strengthening our marriage.

When sexuality is not a struggle. If you do not struggle with sexuality, be grateful for this blessing. Don't assume, however, that you have nothing to work through because of it. Those who enjoy sexuality may not see it with God's eyes.

If you feel you are not a pure person when you have a relationship with your spouse, you may struggle with the opposite side of the problem. It is very virtuous to have a sexual relationship with you husband. You might want to apply the first suggestion in this section. Don't pretend everything is okay. Examine your feelings about sexuality and discuss them with your spouse.

Pray with your spouse about your sexual relationship. Invite the Lord into your partnership to learn how He feels about sexual relationships. He will help you see yourself as he wants you to view yourself in your marriage.

The most important thing I've learned about sexual relations with my companion is that it is good to have a sexual relationship. God has ordained it. As with other areas of our life, our weaknesses can become our strengths.

Conclusion:

1. Many abuse victims have problems with sexuality because their abuse was sexual.

2. God has ordained sexuality in marriage and called it good.

3. Being honest and prayerful with your spouse will help you to resolve this issue and find the joy that comes from a sexual relationship.

WHAT A SPOUSE CAN DO TO HELP

There are many ways a spouse or friend can be helpful

in the healing process. I have listed a few things my husband, Brian, did to help me during my healing.

- He believed in my healing process.

- He was a part of my therapy. He went willingly to support and learn.

- He was willing to change his own unhealthy behavior. (Brian believes everyone has some dysfunction in his life, some people just have more than others. But even those that have less dysfunctional behavior could improve their lives with some type of therapy.)

- He didn't try to make me better. He gave me support and perspective. Then he listened, listened, listened as I discovered a road to healing.

- He didn't act like he had all the answers.

- He helped in practical ways. He was available to pray with me, to listen as I talked, to take over parenting and household demands at various times so I could write in my journal, go to therapy, spend time processing and working through pain and healing issues.

- He believed I could heal completely and wouldn't give up until I did.

- He believed I was doing my best to function on the highest level amidst the pain.

- He believed my heart and spirit were of great worth to God and that God would be there for me.

- He helped me see God's hand in my life.

- He was realistic in his expectations of me. He didn't expect me to be able to have a sexual relationship when I was going through some stages of healing.

- He learned not to initiate a sexual relationship. He was able to acquire an attitude of caring for me rather than simply meet his own needs.

- He tried to show a loving, concerned attitude and kept close to me in his heart when he knew we could not be close sexually. He kept this attitude even when sexual activity was months in waiting. (He says he often chewed fence posts.)

- He accepted when sexuality didn't happen, but kept a hope and belief that one day it would be worth the sacrifice. (He says it has been worth it.)

- He didn't expect me to have dinner ready, the house clean or the errands run. He was grateful when I was able to do these things. He focused on what I did, not what I didn't do.

- He learned to function in the relationship based on where I was that day.

Lessons learned from my husband. Because he cared for me by allowing me freedom from painful activities in our relationship that stemmed from me trying to heal from trauma, we now are able to have a joyful marriage. His sacrifice of sexual activity, his increased work as a partner, his giving more than appeared to be necessary has been a catalyst to my healing. I learned:

- There are selfless men (as opposed to my previous experience).

> *Aug. 10, 1994. My love for Brian grows every day and I am beginning to see more clearly what realistic god-like love is. My husband treats me like a queen. I want to work harder at overcoming my selfish ways and give him the love and goodness he deserves.*
>
> *Brian is becoming more real as a person to me. I have always struggled to see men as gentle, loving people. Every day, by his gentleness and example of Christlike behavior, Brian teaches me what a man of God is like. Our sacred love begins to blossom in such a way that I feel overwhelmed with disbelief at the goodness and love of God.*

- I could trust my spouse. His desires were pure and his focus wasn't on temporary fulfillment but lasting happiness.

- I could believe in him to lead our family in righteousness.

- He deemed me worthy for peace and good. This helped me to begin to treat myself as though I had worth.

- He truly loved me with an unending love. He was willing to give his caring, his sacrifice, his loyalty to me. I could learn to love myself because of his love.

My husband was my greatest ally, my deepest friend, my truest companion, my eternal love. I healed much quicker than it appeared I could because of his patience in long suffering, his faith in my abilities, his encouragement that I could do it. My love for him is deep because he taught me by example and precept what a truly good person is like.

Brian is humble and teachable. He learned and allowed me to be in control of sexuality while I searched to know whether I was acting on what was good for me or what I felt bad for not giving in the past. He helped me to be honest with myself and with him.

Inner child sexuality. We learned we were not always alone in our sexual relationship. When I would shake, wince, be non-responsive or emotionless, this was when the inner child was present being abused again. Brian felt like a perpetrator to this inner part and would feel sickened to do anything. He wanted to help me heal not continue to surface the abuse.

For months when I was deeply into painful memories and issues, Brian gained a new frame of mind. He said when you get married you see a green light to sexuality. Then when you find your wife is full of pain, it is like she is stalled in the middle of the intersection. You put up your own red light so you don't collide with her. When all seems to be better, you cautiously yield until you are given to understand that you again have a green light. There may be multiple times you go back to a red light, then later move again to yield. "Yield" means you move cautiously; you slowly move forward.

As I learned more about my inner child, we were able to put the inner turmoil in safe, non-threatening places before sexuality so my inner children were in a nurturing environment as we had our personal time.

My inner children loved Brian and wanted to be near him because of his care and concern for their pain. He cried with sweet sorrow as my inner children integrated and said goodbye. (See *Parenting the Inner Child, p. 123.)*

You can learn how to support your companion by going to therapy alone and with your spouse. Seek all the knowledge you can to learn about the pain. As you learn to master yourself, you can be a support by freely giving your strength to bless your sweetheart's life.

You may never learn to be the perfect spouse as your companion heals, but with every effort you can learn, overcome weakness, and give support. Your help will be remembered and will assist healing in a lasting way.

CHAPTER FIVE

AS I AM KNOWN THROUGH GOD'S CLEAR GLASS

"Yet thou hast said, I know thee by name, and thou hast also found grace in my sight.

"Now therefore, I pray thee, if I have found grace in thy sight, shew me now thy way, that I may know thee, that I may find grace in thy sight" (Exodus 33:12-13).

Victims of childhood trauma often feel ostracized from where they long to be. They wonder where God is. They may ask, "How does God view me from His clear glass as my inner self reflects back to Him? Is the darkened chaos I see in my inner child worthy of His love? How can He help me understand my past experiences and child within?"

Do you wonder when you will feel the grace God has for you? How do you accept and know God as He sends love from heaven? How do you feel your goodness as you see through God's eyes? Do you understand your innocence and accept gifts of strength? Do you see only a blur between you and God?

You may say, "I long to know myself as God knows me."

SPIRITUAL CONFUSION

Why am I unable to apply scriptural truths?
Why do I feel as though I am unable to move
forward?

Sin causes spiritual confusion, even if the person in confusion did not commit the sin. A perpetrator's sin can encompass an abuse victim in dark confusion. The sin affects the victim's ability to see, recognize, and follow the light from the Savior.

You may be in spiritual darkness because of the sins and unrighteous traditions of your family. You have experienced the dark sins of an evil act perpetrated upon you. You may have learned unrighteous traditions in your family or you may have interpreted your family lifestyle since the abuse with a distorted perspective. You may have believed untruths the perpetrator said and did which created spiritual confusion.

A mudslide to your soul. Imagine your body as a house with many windows. If there was a tremendous storm and a mud slide engulfed the house, mud would cover the windows. Even after the storm was over, light could not permeate the mud-covered windows. Sometimes shades of light might be distinguished, but they would be dim and you would not be able to clearly see the beautiful trees, birds, flowers, and sky.

You would still be in darkness. Your perception of the world would be dark, lonely, and distorted. The abuser's act is like a mud slide to your soul--spiritual light is distorted.

The mud didn't come because the house was bad; it came because mud happens. The house is completely worthy to have windows full of light, but it will take some work to dig the house out of the mud and fix it up. The house did nothing wrong, it is a perfectly acceptable home.

The inner part of yourself has experienced deep darkness while in childhood. The abused child is unable to interpret and process the painful traumatic experiences. The abuse caused numbness, confusing feelings, and guilt. Darkness continues because of pain. All are effects of the sin of another.

Spiritual confusion continues because of inability to recognize light coming in. Truth is distorted. You were not able to comprehend the evil darkness as a child. You were restricted by childlike thinking. "When I was a child, I spake as a child, I understood as a child, I thought as a child" (1 Cor. 13:11).

So as a child you did nothing with the abuse experience except endure and survive. Now as an adult in order to be whole you are invited to work through the pain and confusion of your childlike inner self so that light will permeate your life.

"See[ing] through a glass darkly." "For now we see through a glass, darkly; but then face to face: now I know in part; but then shall I know even as also I am known" (v.12).

As you heal you will be capable of true progression that will come because of being whole spiritually. Light will come into your life and you will be able to see yourself, gospel truths, and eternity more clearly. You will discover who you really are. Instead of a pile of mud, you will see a beautiful house of God.

"And now abideth faith, hope, charity, these three; but the greatest of these is charity" (v.13). Charity is the pure love and pure light of Christ that shines forth through darkness. If you allow the Savior to help you dig yourself out of darkness into light, you will then be full of love to others and long to help them find this great light. This is charity. Your faith and hope will lead you to this light and this charity.

Letting the light in. There are various ways to

receive light as you work through healing. Here are a few suggestions:

- Talk to trusted friends or church clergy. Tell them what you need. Ask them to help you by listening, supporting, praying, and learning to understand your trials. (See *Receiving Help from Others, p. 143.*)
- Ask others to pray for you.
- Seek professional counseling. (See *Should I Go to Therapy? p. 77.*)

- Study the scriptures. Read scriptures about pain or hope, suffering or sorrow. The study topics are endless. The scriptures can be a "lamp unto [your] feet, and a light unto [your] path" (Psalms 119:105).

You are perfectly acceptable to God. Light will flow through you again, but it will take work on your part to receive the light. The mud--or act of another--was not pleasing to God and He will help you fix things if you invite Him to be a part your healing.

Conclusion:
1. You may be in spiritual confusion because of evil inflicted on you as a child.
2. This darkness comes partly because you were young when you experienced abuse. You may be dealing with the experience with childlike thinking from the time of the experience.
3. The darkness didn't happen because you are bad.
4. God will help you bring light back into your life.

FEELING ABANDONED BY GOD
Why didn't God help me when I needed him?
Why doesn't God help me now?

Abuse victims feel abandoned by God. The chains of
sins placed around them by their perpetrator feel too heavy to
remove by themselves, but victims don't feel like they receive
assistance from their Savior. They may believe in God, but do
not believe He is there to help them. They may believe He
forsook them when they needed Him as a child. It's hard to
believe He will help now.

Feeling God has forsaken you. When you go
through trials, it is important to feel you can turn to God for
help. When children are abused, they may cry from their heart
for help. When help doesn't come, they start to believe that
even God who knows everything will not help them when they
need it. They start to believe they cannot turn to God to receive
help because help doesn't come.

Abuse victims may echo the cry of the children of
Israel, "The Lord hath forsaken me, and my Lord hath forgotten
me" (Isaiah 49:14).

God has not forsaken you, but you may have felt
abandoned because God did not step in and stop your abuse
even when you were pleading for that to happen. God does not
thwart someone else's agency even if that person's actions will
cause pain.

Exercising agency. We live life to experience the joys
of living. As we do this we also experience pain and sadness
that come because people choose how they will act or exercise
their agency. God does not take away agency. He allows His
children to act and then consequences follow. (See *Why We*

Experience Suffering, Pain, and Sorrow, p. 296; The Savior's Suffering, Pain, and Sorrow [The Atonement], p. 306.)

I feel God says, "There are some things I don't do because of agency, but I do owe you healing. I will help you heal. As you pray and seek for what I promised to do, I will freely give those things to you."

God will not do anything that takes away adult choices or someone's agency. Therefore, you may not receive answers to prayers that interfere with another's agency. But you may ask for knowledge about how to change your circumstances. You can ask for understanding, strength, and endurance.

God will give you ability to comprehend His ways, insight to better understand a hardship, and wisdom to know how to overcome. He can give you relief from pain. God can also to help you understand your value and know how to apply His word. There are many other things you can ask that God will freely give line upon line according to your growth and His will.

God works within boundaries of truth. As you learn and understand God's ways you will see how to seek and receive God's help. He is there and His arm is reached out to receive you and give you blessings you can't even imagine.

Conclusion:

1. Victims felt betrayed by God in the past and feel He won't be available for present needs.

2. God is there for you and will help you. You must learn how to seek Him.

3. When you learn about exercising agency, you can better trust God.

NO ONE WILL SAVE ME; WHERE IS MY SAVIOR?

Why didn't anyone protect me?
Why am I so angry with my mother?

Most victims of abuse have "mother" issues, if not entire family issues. They feel hurt and abandoned by their family, or at least their mother. They wonder why their family didn't somehow know and save them from abuse.

As children they may not have even known they needed to be saved, but as an adult they realize what the sinful acts of another have done to their life. They search desperately for answers as to why no one was there to "clasp this child out of the bands of hell" at the time of the abuse.

Where is my mother? When I was going through so much pain, I experienced flashbacks that brought back memories of my abuse. I looked at what happened crying, "Someone help me! Who can help? Please, someone help my baby--me!"

Then I would think, "My mother! Where is my mother? Doesn't she love me? Doesn't she care about me? Won't she save me?!"

Mothers are our first contact in this world. Our mother is the one we knew intimately even before life begins. We look to our mother to save us, to be there when we need something, to hold us when we cry, to make our pains all better, to save us. We think, *If our mother doesn't care enough to be there for us, who will?*

To a child's mind, a mother knows everything. She knows if we put our underwear on backwards without even looking for the tag. How could she not know to save her child who is being abused?

Feb. 12, 1989. My sister, Kaye, brought to my attention the lack in my relationship with Mom. I have not been very open and loving to Mom, and as a person I don't even really know her. I think it is worth my time and prayerful effort to repent of this and work towards improving our relationship. I have been deeply critical and have had overwhelmingly high expectations of her. I forget to let her have a break.

Abuse is quiet. Abuse may <u>never</u> be talked about by the abuser and a child doesn't feel permitted to say anything. She feels frightened to tell anyone about what is happening. I remember thinking that sexual abuse was a normal experience. I thought all men abused and everyone knew they did, but they just wouldn't talk about it.

When I was five, I went to the school to get my eyes checked. The doctor took me behind a curtain for the exam. I assumed he would abuse me because we were in a private place. I was surprised that he did not. I thought abuse was an everyday experience and could come from anyone.

Sexuality is meant to be private. It was given to Adam and Eve as a private part of their relationship. Children feel the innate private-ness of sexuality. From the perpetrator's actions or words, they understand the rule not to talk about the abuse. The perpetrator may or may not tell the child, "Don't tell your mommy," but the silence during the abuse says it all. You don't talk.

Some children may try to talk, but they lack the vocabulary to give details. The adult may not recognize that the child is trying to talk about sexuality. Unless adults are prepared to realize that abuse could happen to a child, they most likely will not recognize any signs of abuse. There is no experience from the past that prepares them. (See *Recognizing Signs of Abuse, p. 53*.)

We need a Savior. Regardless of whether a mother or family member is capable of recognizing the abuse, children need someone to save them. The mother is only human. She has her own needs, weaknesses, limitations, pain, and sin. She cannot save her children from the world.

Sometimes a mother may fail you, but the Savior never will. He promises, "Can a woman forget her sucking child, that she should not have compassion on the son of her womb? yea, they may forget, yet will I not forget thee.

"Behold, I have graven thee upon the palms of my hands" (Isaiah 49:15-16).

I long to save my children from every trial and pain in this world, but I can't. I know my mother, too, would have wanted to be there to care for me, nurture me, teach me, and especially to have stopped the abuse. I believe most mothers would. But others are not our Saviors. Christ is the only Savior. "Neither is salvation in any other: for there is none other name under heaven given among men, whereby we must be saved" (Acts 4:12).

The child self does not know or understand God's sacrifice for us. Your adult self must teach the inner child who the Savior is, what He has done, and how to receive His mercy.

We grieve that our mothers and others did not save us. Even if they could have stopped the abuse soon after it started, they could not heal what the abuse did. They could only support us as we heal. Complete healing comes only through the Savior.

We need our Savior. He longs for us to make His Atonement real in our lives. I love Him for every step of healing. I know He is my only Savior. I have faith you can discover for yourself what I have come to know.

Conclusion:

1. Many abuse victims feel abandoned or neglected by their mother or other family members who might have rescued them.

2. Abuse is quiet and private. This keeps many people from seeing the signs that might alert them to the abuse.

3. While we want our mother or some other adult care giver to rescue us, the only person who can save us is our Savior.

FEELING GOD DOES NOT LOVE ME

Why does God bless other people and He doesn't care about me?

Why don't I deserve God's blessings?

Abuse victims may recognize God's hand in the lives of other people. They may pray for God to bless others, but not themselves because they do not feel His love. They feel they are not deserving of God's love.

What keeps you from feeling God's love? You do not feel peace and understanding from God because pain gets in the way of your capacity to recognize God's love. When you are full of pain, you feel overloaded with numbness, anger, guilt, or confusion. These intense feelings sabotage your ability to feel other emotions.

You may find it difficult to feel the still small voice of peace from God. Even though He sends messages, you may not recognize them because you hear the effects of childhood emotions and trauma screaming within yourself.

What do we want from God? We want to feel His love. God's "hand is stretched out" (Isa. 5:25), but we cannot receive from Him or anyone else. We feel anger or guilt but are unable to feel the opposite--peace.

God promises, "I will not leave you comfortless: I will come to you" (John 14:18). God promises love and protection, but even if we see His help we don't feel His promises fulfilled.

As you keep moving toward healing, you will be able to receive God's love and help. But there is no room to receive when you are full of so much emotion. You are trapped within these emotions and must be able to find a way for them to be released. As you work through your emotions, purge them, and give the pain to God, you will be able to feel His sweet blessings--His love.

Nov. 14, 1982. Today is a great day! I feel pretty good about myself and what I'm doing with my life. It was funny how for such a long time I couldn't get the spirit of pure love for the gospel. I felt so lost just wondering who I was. Now I sort of see the light. I really love being close to God. The hardest thing is taking the first step.

Thank you Father, for putting a spark of light in my heart and a piece of "I-can-do-it" in my today and tomorrow, I love you, Julie.

Rescue from pain. You may feel God does not love you because He doesn't remove your pain. You feel you must deserve the pain. You may want God to release you from your pain to show His love to you, but God won't do this. Removing your pain would take away your agency and rob you of eternal growth. You must work <u>through</u> the pain.

Everyone experiences pain. Even God's Only Begotten Son experienced pain. Did He <u>deserve</u> it? Of course not. Pain does not come only because you deserve it. You are here to gain experience. You may not deserve the pain, but you do deserve the rewards from overcoming. You must put forth energy to receive this reward.

God's love is unconditional. You may think you

210

have to prove your worth to God in order for you to be worthy of His love. God loves you regardless of worthiness. God's love is unconditional.

Children are completely whole and worthy. Your child self, not your adult self, feels she needs to prove her worth. God loves you no matter what you feel you are like. You are His child. (See *The Broken Inner Self, p. 4; What Does God Think of Your Inner Child? p. 215.*)

April, 23, 1995. I learned in church that God's love will not increase as we become better. God loves me completely and I don't have to do anything to earn or lose His love. He will always love me completely and unconditionally no matter what I do. He will not love me more if I am perfect. He will not love me more or less if I sin. He loves me completely. I have written this several ways because it is so hard to comprehend and I'm trying to absorb its meaning to the fullest.

Your child self tells you that you don't deserve the blessings God offers. Your inner child tells you that you don't even deserve answers to your prayers. Others deserve prayers answered, but you don't. You may pray with great faith for others and see prayers answered for them, but can't see prayers answered in your own behalf. If you do have a prayer answered, you don't trust yourself to accept the answer because you feel unworthy. You often discount it because you believe you don't deserve God's kindness in your life.

God does love you. You may not feel it, but His love is there. As you work through your pain it will be easier to feel God's loving influence in your life. Muster the courage to attempt a relationship with your Heavenly Father. Even though your inner child may not <u>feel</u> His love, let your adult self act on

the <u>knowledge</u> that He loves you. (See *Distorted Thinking. p. 13.*)
        Act believing in God's love. As you do this, tell your-
self, "I know God loves me because I have blessings that I can
see--even if I can't feel His love. I will believe and later I will
feel." By doing this, your child self will respond to your
teaching of truth and this will serve as a tool for changing the
inner child's feelings towards truth, thus helping you to heal.

        Conclusion
        1. God's love is there for you, but you may have a
hard time recognizing it because of emotions screaming inside of
you.
        2. God loves you, but He will not remove your pain.
        3. God's love is unconditional. You don't have to
prove your worth to Him.

LOSS OF IDENTITY AS A FOLLOWER OF CHRIST
        *How can I be a child of God? I don't feel love
from God.*
        Should a follower of God feel empty inside?

        Many people in inner turmoil ask, "Who am I?" They
have lost their identity as a follower of Christ. They may feel
estranged from God because they feel He abandoned them.
We are all children of God, but being a child of God is
irrelevant unless you feel like God's child.
        Picture pain and joy on a scale with pain on one end
and joy on the other. You have gone through incredible pain,
but because there is opposition in all things you also have the
potential to experience indescribable joy. The basis of that joy
is discovering who you are. When you truly know you are a
daughter of a Heavenly King who loves you, you can never be

the same. You may have had an abusive earthly father and/or mother, but you can find hope and joy knowing you have a perfect Heavenly Father.

How do you discover God? You may wonder, as Nicodemus did, how you can be born of God. Start out simply. Call on God in faith. Try to believe you have a loving Heavenly Father. Imagine He listens to you and will answer your prayers

You can learn that you are a child of God. It is hard to offer a prayer to an unknown being when you may feel unsure such a being exists. But as you seek to find your Heavenly Father and Jesus Christ, His Son, they will make themselves known to you and you will begin to experience their love.

God has a wonderful gift prepared for you. Once you learn about your Heavenly Father, you are ready to learn about the wonderful gift He has given each of us. God sent His Son, Jesus Christ to earth where He offered Himself as a sacrifice for our sin and pain. He wants us to accept the gift of His Atonement. (See *The Savior's Suffering, Pain, and Sorrow [The Atonement], p. 306.*)

The Savior suffered for the sinner, but I believe His greatest empathy goes to the victim of sin who suffers because there is opposition in the world. Much of the Savior's suffering came because of the wicked acts of others. He knows the pain of being a victim. He experienced unfeeling brutality at the hands of others. He suffered pain beyond all in the Garden of Gethsemane. He knows.

Adam's fall meant mankind would suffer because of sin. The Son of Man atoned for all suffering. By experiencing a degree of the pain He experienced, we then have the capacity to feel the joy the Savior now feels as a result of having overcome all.

Your Father in Heaven wants to help you heal.
Imagine that it is going to take 100% of heaven's work and faith
to get through your healing. I have always felt if I gave 1% to
my healing (which <u>felt</u> like 99-100% to me), Heavenly Father
would make up the rest. If I followed the guidance or light of
Christ, though I couldn't see the end result, my mind would be
enlightened and I would be able to receive growth from God.
God gave 99% after I gave my 1%. You'll see the 99% after
you give 1%. You will see the depth and breadth of all the
Savior has done.

The trick was I had to initiate the healing. I had to be
willing to give by taking the first step. My 1% had to come at
the beginning. I couldn't say, "I'll move forward after I see the
whole picture. Show me what I'll gain, how this will affect my
family, posterity, and eternity and I'll follow thy promptings." I
had to give fearing I might be giving up all, but believing that I
was following God.

*Aug. 5, 1994. Today is my 30th birthday and I want
to write how I feel about life. I am happy to be turning 30.
I am happy about where my life is now and the potential for
growth and learning that lies ahead.*

*Everyone has trials to face in this life but God is
there to help us find peace, growth and learning. We can
choose if those trials will improve or destroy our spiritual
growth.*

*I know that God loves me but He does not provide
an easy road. He expects work, sacrifice, and faith on my
part and after <u>all I can do</u> He will make up <u>all</u> of the difference. The Savior atoned to make up the difference, to
allow us every possible chance, but there are no shortcuts,*

no easy roads and no excuses for not doing our part. Blessings do not come without doing all we can.

I have noticed as I repent, read, pray, and try, my heart is softer and I am easier to mold and work with.

I love God. I thank Him for loving me enough to give me situations that cause me to grow. God knows what it's going to take for me to become like Him. I am going to work at becoming soft enough that He may work with me.

You can learn that you are a child of God. As you seek to know God, He will reveal Himself to you. You will feel the love He has for you, His precious child.

Conclusion:

1. Many abuse victims lose their identity as a child of God.

2. To feel joy, you need to internalize the knowledge that you are a child of God.

3. God offers the gift of the Atonement to all His children through His Son, Jesus Christ.

4. Exercising faith in God will help you learn you are God's child.

WHAT DOES GOD THINK OF YOUR INNER CHILD?

Does God care about children?
What would the Savior do to help my inner child?

Jesus loves little children. When He lived on earth He spent time with little children. He taught adults to become like little children. He felt great sorrow as He watched you experience abuse as a child.

Jesus values little children. Jesus showed how He valued children during his life on earth.

"Then were there brought unto him little children, that he should put his hands on them, and pray: and the disciples rebuked them.

"But Jesus said, Suffer little children, and forbid them not, to come unto me: for of such is the kingdom of heaven.

"And he laid his hands on them, and departed thence" (Matthew 19:13-15).

Jesus had much to do as He set up His kingdom on earth. He knew He did not have much time but He wanted to spend time with little children.

Jesus knew the worth of little children and taught, "Take heed that ye despise not one of these little ones; for I say unto you, that in heaven their angels do always behold the face of my Father which is in heaven" (Matt. 18:10).

The Savior wants children to come to Him. Little children must have a Savior or they will be forever in pain. Your inner child is counting on you to lead her to the Savior. She doesn't know how to get to Him by herself. The Savior blessed and healed the children when their parents sought the Savior or brought their children to Him. You must learn to parent your inner child by bringing her to Christ to be blessed and healed. (See *Parenting the Inner Child, p. 123.*)

There were times I was suffering and felt the pains of the child within. I taught her I was there to protect her. I taught her she was good and innocent but I was helpless to take away the pain of what had happened. She needed the Savior to be healed.

In my mind's eye I would imagine the child of my youth with the Savior. I went to Him taking her to receive help from Him. The most precious moments of my healing were when

within myself I saw the Savior come and hold my child. I felt
His incredible power of healing and His unspeakable love. I felt
the precious embrace of a merciful Savior who had given His all
so I might live.

All of my inner children believed in the Savior's divinity.
He alone has the capacity to heal us. Your child who was
abused doesn't know how to internalize the goodness of God.
You must embrace and teach her so her wounds can be bound,
her eyes of understanding can be healed, and her broken heart
can be mended by the Only Begotten Son.

Conclusion:
1. Jesus loves little children.
2. Teach your inner child to trust and love the Savior
so she can be healed.

HOW DOES GOD ASK YOUR ADULT SELF TO VIEW YOUR INNER CHILD?

*What should I do if I can't accept the inner child
concept?*

*What am I supposed to do with my painful inner
child?*

Adults have a role to be an example and to patiently
teach correct principles so children will learn to govern themselves. Children (especially teenagers) respond to sincere,
loving, and honest guidance. They rebel or feel ostracized when
they are forced, manipulated, taught dishonestly, coerced, or
given harsh judgment.

You have an inner child (or children) that must be taught
correct principles at her developmental level. To do this you
must learn how to view your inner child. This can be difficult. I

resisted the concept of an inner child. The concept seemed uncomfortable, foreign, even unacceptable. When I fought her existence, I hurt myself. When I worked with her, I progressed. As I came to love her, I healed.

Adults are responsible to teach their children. Children must be taught correct principles. "Train up a child in the way he should go: and when he is old, he will not depart from it" (Proverbs 22:6). If children are not taught, the parents are responsible. As you befriend and parent the inner child, you can safely guide her to the Father and Son.

Children learn from their environment and the examples of others. They then live as they have learned. If a child is not taught, her actions are on the shoulders of those who should have taught her.

Work to be filled with love for little children. If you have faith, hope, and charity (the love of God), you will know and see as God sees your inner child. There is no evil in your inner child, her nature is pure. When you are filled with charity, which is everlasting love; you will love little children with a perfect love. As you strive to be a true follower of the Savior, your adult self will be filled with charity, the pure love of Christ. Then you can see your inner child as she is, worthy of salvation.

God promises, "For I am the Lord, I change not" (Malachi 3:6). God is trustworthy. He doesn't change. He is just, merciful, and omnipotent. You can believe what He says. If in the past God said He valued children, this is still true today.

What is your responsibility towards your inner child? The Lord expects you to care for the children. I feel Jesus says to adults, look at your responsibility to be an example of me, to teach, to love, and to nurture. Your inner children are dependent on your adult self to lead the way to the Savior. It is ominous to think of the damage that has been done in those tender years. Some inner children may not seem lovable or easily understood because of this. Your unconditional love is critical because you must deal with their outward expression of pain.

The Savior loves little children and it is your opportunity to assist the Savior by teaching and nurturing your own inner child. There will be many who can assist you, but you must learn and apply truth and lead her to Christ's healing through your example. Christ's healing power is awe provoking beyond our ability to comprehend.

What happens if your inner child has been taught false principles? You must have the courage to embrace and teach your inner child pure truth to correct lies so darkness will not continue. Otherwise you will give your pain to others, and your heart will be hardened. Truth not applied is truth rejected.

God loves you and wants you to teach your inner child at her developmental level. As she learns the ways of the Savior (which is truth), He can bless her with His atoning love. (See *Erikson Chart p. 5; Parenting the Inner Child, p. 123.*)

As you care for your inner child, loving her as the Savior would, you are promised the blessing of peace. "And all thy children shall be taught of the Lord; and great shall be the peace of thy children" (Isaiah 54:13).

You can show Christlike love when you embrace your inner child as the Savior embraced children who came to Him. You must teach your sweet and innocent inner child and show her the way back to the Savior.

Your inner child can teach you. Children are pure

vessels that the Savior enables to teach adults. Your inner child
needs to teach you about what formed the person you are so
you can become the person God plans for you to become. The
inner child is there because of heaven's miracle to enable you to
survive. She understands truth you may not know and cannot
access without her.

My inner children were a blessing to me. Their example
taught my adult self to come unto Christ. They who submitted
to imperfect care givers were hurt. Learning from them, I submitted to the omnipotent caregiver, then taught and nurtured
them guiding them toward healing. The Savior blessed them to
gain eternal peace.

Conclusion:
1. We are to look at our inner child as pure and
innocent.
2. We must love our inner child, teach her, and guide
her to the Savior. As we teach and love the inner child, she will
teach us.

GUILT

Why do I feel so unworthy?
How can I get over feeling that if only I had done
something different, the abuse would not have happened?

Most abuse victims feel guilty. They feel they were
responsible for the abuse or they could have done something to
prevent it from happening. They may think, *If only I would*
have. . . or *Why did I go there?* or *I should have known.*
They may feel unworthy and act on those feelings or they
overcompensate and become a chronic "repenter."

Imagine someone hurting another. The person first

thinks about the act, then crystallizes the thought as hands turn thought into action. As the person acts, hurting someone, the pain is given to the victim. The victim or child internalizes a feeling of responsibility and guilt as she tries to make sense of a helpless feeling.

Is guilt ever useful? We need to feel we have power over what happens to us. We need hope. Feeling guilt is a survival technique. It kept us alive as a child and helped us feel hope. Children accept guilt for what happened and leave the perpetrator innocent. Being willing to take the weight on themselves makes their world safe.

For example, imagine a child is playing and Auntie spanks the child violently for no reason. Will the child think, *Auntie hurt me and I didn't do anything wrong. Auntie made a bad choice.* Or will the child think, *I must have done something wrong. I don't know what it is, but I need to do better so Auntie won't hurt me again.*

The child will most probably feel guilty because she hopes she can stop the hurtful action by acting differently. Without hope we have nothing. This displaced guilt saves the child from despair and helps her hope for a better world.

The guilt that was useful during childhood is harmful as an adult. It can stop you from feeling worthy, from seeing your innocence, and from embracing and teaching your inner child truth. Guilt can stop you from seeing what truly happened. Guilt can make you feel evil. If you feel you are bad, you see no reason to refrain from becoming immoral, an alcoholic, a lesbian. These distorted views could feed into acting out how you feel about yourself.

I was guilt-ridden as this journal entry shows.

June 21, 1986. I WILL BE A BETTER PERSON! As

I live the gospel, set goals and pray I will be at peace with myself, the world, and what happens around me. As I look for the good I WILL FIND IT.

I am so ashamed of my weaknesses, of my unchristian thoughts and actions. I want to be more <u>worthy</u>. BUT I WON'T GIVE UP! NO MATTER HOW MANY TIMES I FALL, I WILL HOLD ON AND STAND AGAIN. I pray for this.

Some who feel they are bad will act the way they feel, hoping to make sense of their feelings. They feel they might as well act the way they feel they are. Others who feel they are bad will work to conquer that feeling, believing that if they become good enough--the good will drown out the feelings of guilt. They believe being extra good will conquer evil.

These kinds of feelings may lead to problems with perfectionism. Some will feel so helpless about the way they feel they want to end their life. (See *Kohlberg Chart, p. 11; Perfectionism, p. 27.*)

How do you eliminate guilt? You talk or write about what happened to you and the feelings associated with what happened. As you talk and write about what happened, your adult self will eventually see that the child self could not have stopped or known how to prevent the abuse.

You teach yourself or have others help teach you that the perpetrator chose wrong. You were not in the wrong. You start to see that your actions were free from sin.

Mar. 25, 1995. I have wondered about my responsibility and/or guilt related to the abuse. Yesterday I woke with a question in my mind, "During or before your abuse, did you ever feel a prompting or warning from the Holy

Ghost that you were choosing the wrong thing?"

My answer was, "I know what it feels like to be warned by the Holy Ghost before sin is committed. No, I never felt this. I only felt vulnerable, trapped, and in danger. I never made a decision because I didn't really know I had a choice to be somewhere else."

This morning at 2:30 a.m. I awoke from a dream. My dream deepened my understanding of my childhood innocence. I dreamed about being in an abusive situation. When I turned around, I was Kati, my 2-year-old daughter. This dream caused me to feel and see the way I really was-- innocent. Kati could never be responsible for abuse and would never deserve such treatment, no matter what she'd done or could do mistakenly. She is an innocent child.

You may have heard the story of a little boy who was riding his tricycle by his home in a big city. He ran into an electric pole with his tricycle just as the power went out throughout the entire city. For many years he felt responsible for this act. He believed he had caused the black out.

Years later still feeling bad, he finally told someone his painful secret. Only then was he able to see that it would have been impossible for him to have caused the outage. Telling his story to someone relieved him of his feelings of guilt and opened his eyes to see the situation from an adult point of view.

When you get your fearful secret out in the open, you can examine it through logical adult eyes. You see more clearly what happened. Distorted ideas, like guilt for another's actions, can be stripped away.

You can gain relief as you teach your inner child about her innocence. As you recognize your innocence, you can overcome your need for perfectionism which is simply a mechanism you created to deal with guilt. You won't feel the need to repent any more for someone else's sin. You will be freed from bondage.

Instead of feeling hopeless now you can teach truths that will give your inner child the hope she had no resources to obtain in her youth. What a relief!

Conclusion:
1. Guilt gives hope to the child, but holds the adult back.
2. The perpetrator, not the child, is guilty for the abuse.
3. Talking or writing about the abuse will help you better understand what really happened.

SHAME

Why do I feel embarrassed for something that wasn't my fault?

If I feel shame, does it mean I was in the wrong?

Shame is usually guilt's companion. Ironic as it may be, the innocent victim feels shame and the guilty party does not. Being exploited brings feelings of shame because you internalize the guilt of the sin placed upon you. Women who have been raped often report feeling shame. Shame is a normal feeling that occurs when you have no control over an abuser's wrongdoing.

Feeling shamed is normal for those who have been sinned upon. It stems from feelings of helplessness when you witnessed evil or helplessly experienced evil. Shame is not a sign you have done wrong even though you were treated as though you were bad.

When you are abused, the abuser instills a feeling that the fault was yours. (You asked for it or you wanted the perpetrator to do it.) The perpetrator may tell you that you are evil or deserve the act happening to you.

Why do the righteous feel shame?   The righteous feel shame to even speak of secret and dark acts, "For it is a shame even to speak of those things which are done of them in secret" (Eph. 5:12). Shame is feeling embarrassed for experiencing humiliation. It is the feeling of being treated far much less than you are worth. You were treated worse than how animals treat their offspring.

An abused person feels below others because she has been treated inhumanely. She feels unworthy to look people in the eye, feeling they will know what happened to her. She feels the perpetrator's evil actions represent what she is worth. Being shamed strips feelings of self worth.

Feb. 6, 1983. My Father, oh how I beg Thee to forgive me for all my imperfections. Bless me to have the strength to repent for all that I am ashamed of and never do them again. Bless me to become the best me I can be. I want Thee to be proud of me. Please forgive me for the past and bless me to strive to be better.

Why does the inner child feel shame? The inner child's role is to testify. The inner child experienced the abuse and carries it for you while you try to help her heal. You might say to the inner child, "Thou hast known my reproach, and my shame, and my dishonour: mine adversaries are all before thee" (Ps. 69:19).

Now, unlike during your childhood, you are capable of being the leader and teacher of life's experiences. You can show your inner child how to feel great worth instead of shame. As an adult you hold the power to instill goodness or evil in the child self. Children are the product of the good or evil taught to them.

When will the wicked feel shame? Even if the wicked never feel shame in this life, they will feel shame when they stand before God after the resurrection. They will be brought to stand with shame and awful guilt before the bar of God. Job wrote, "They that hate thee shall be clothed with shame; and the dwelling place of the wicked shall come to nought" (Job 8:22).

What does the Savior teach about shame? It is important to understand the difference between guilt and shame. You feel guilt when you do evil or think you've done evil. You feel shame because evil was done. You may also be shamed by others if you do things they do not see as true. (See *Telling the Secret, p. 163*.)

The Savior felt the shame of the world. People did not understand Him and His mission. He felt all of the evil acts that the human race did. He willingly experienced the shame of it all. "I gave my back to the smiters, and my cheeks to them that plucked off the hair: I hid not my face from shame and spitting" (Isa. 50:6).

Christ's apostles rejoiced when they suffered shame in Christ's name. "And they departed from the presence of the council, rejoicing that they were counted worthy to suffer shame for his name" (Acts 5:41).

The Savior knows what it feels to be shamed. He taught us to overcome shame through endurance which will lead to being exalted. "Looking unto Jesus the author and finisher of our faith; who for the joy that was set before him endured the cross, despising the shame, and is set down at the right hand of the throne of God" (Heb. 12:2).

You are promised the same blessing. If you believe in

the Holy One of Israel, and endure your personal crosses of the world, and despise the shame of it, you will inherit the kingdom of God, which was prepared from the foundation of the world. Then your joy will be full forever.

How do you overcome shame? Imagine you are attacked in a dark parking lot. You feel embarrassed and ashamed about what happened to you. You don't want anyone to see you are vulnerable and hurt.

You don't want anyone to see what happened to you. Your arm is broken, but you try to heal by yourself rather than going to the doctor. You can survive, but you may lose the use of your arm.

Later, if you go to the doctor, the doctor will have to reset the arm to allow it to heal. You may have to have physical therapy for it to function properly. But, because of what the doctor knows, he can make the arm usable again. The doctor knows what to do to help the arm heal. The victim with her lack of knowledge doesn't have the ability to fix the arm so it can heal properly. (See *Willingness to Heal, p. 58.*)

Freedom from shame. God wants you freed from your abuser's acts. The perpetrator will ultimately feel shame for the act, not you. Imagine yourself giving the shame to him. The feeling of shame is real, but you can learn to give it to the one who deserves it. Look to the truth about who is going to hold whom back. You don't deserve to suffer because of the abuser's bitter acts.

In order to heal you must quit hiding your broken self and allow someone to help you. The Savior, a prayerfully chosen therapist, and others know how to help you heal your broken heart and clear up the darkness from your soul.

Just as a person who is attacked should not let shame

keep her from receiving help, so you too should not let another person's act hold you back. You need support and care to set your life toward healing.

"Fear not, for thou shalt not be ashamed: neither be thou confounded, for thou shalt not be put to shame: for thou shalt forget the shame of thy youth" (Isa. 54:4).

You can heal from the "shame of [your] youth." You can look to the Savior as an example of one who was innocent who conquered shame. You will overcome your feelings of shame as you bring them out in the open and allow yourself to heal and find joy.

Conclusion:

1. Righteous people feel shame when they experience evil. Even the Savior felt shame.

2. If you endure shame, you will join your Heavenly Father and be exalted with Him.

3. Although you feel shame from your abuse, you need to come out of hiding so you can receive help to heal.

WHAT ENSURES YOU AS A CHILD DID NOT SIN?

Can little children sin?
Are children basically bad?

Many people believe that when children come to this earth they need to be cleansed from the sins of our original parents, Adam and Eve. They do not believe that children come to this earth clean and pure. They do not understand that children are not accountable for their actions when they are little.

While majoring in Child Development, I was taught that children are not evil and they act as they are taught. To some extent, they are products of those around them. I was shocked as I internalized the concept that sin forms untrue beliefs in children. Children though full of light themselves, take in darkness because of adult sin. The darkness continues through childhood and into adulthood.

Children are whole and cannot commit sin. Even though children may have been taught untruths, are they sinful? The scriptures give insight:

The disciples asked who was the greatest in the kingdom. Jesus called a child to him saying, "Except ye be converted, and become as little children, ye shall not enter into the kingdom of heaven" (Matthew 18:3).

The Savior is teaching that children are pure and without sin. He goes on to say, "And whoso shall receive one such little child in my name receiveth me" (v. 5). The Savior did not come to teach that children were evil. He blessed them.

Children are not capable of repenting because they are not capable of sinning. They think as a child. Their mind cannot comprehend evil well enough to be responsible for the consequences of their actions.

Little children are innocent and need no repentance. To believe your inner child can sin and has need to repent is to have no hope of a just God. Children need no judgment and have no need for repentance. They are encompassed within the mercy of the Savior's Atonement. The Savior's Atonement covers all the need for mercy and justice in the world.

If you think the inner child sinned, you will treat her as though she is guilty of wickedness. This will condemn you because your actions will teach your inner child she is evil when she isn't. You will deny her the full ability to learn truth freely, to gain a testimony of how the Savior's Atonement works, and ultimately to heal. You will condemn yourself because when your adult self denies the inner child an opportunity to heal, you deny yourself hope to heal.

Your inner child is looking for freedom from darkness. If you tell her she is responsible for the darkness inside her she will be angry or try to repent to rid herself of the darkness. She cannot find light in this untruth. She is to be loved, taught, and guided to truth, healing, and her Savior.

Adults choose the truths and traditions they'll embrace. As an adult, you choose if you'll continue the beliefs or traditions of your fathers. You decide if you will embrace more information. As you seek truth, you too evaluate if you have all the light available to you from God. You choose if you want to become more than you were given. You decide whether to throw out the darkness or lies of your youth. This is the agency of adulthood.

If adults do not choose to seek and live truth, they will not gain attributes of a child and will remain in darkness seeing distortions in life around them. Their inner children will be treated with little worth, goodness, or understanding because of these distortions.

Adults come to Christ differently than the way children come to Him. The adult self repents to come to Christ, but the inner child learns she is a child of God to be able to come to Christ. All adults sin, but children are engulfed in the Savior's mercy.

What is the goal of the adult? To be under the law (accountable) and become like little children. If you act as you were taught, by unrighteous example or precept, you become a natural man or woman. So learning truth through the Holy

Ghost and following it is vital. If you yield to the enticings of the Holy Spirit, He will guide you to become childlike. (See *Following the Direction of the Holy Spirit, p. 234.*)

Your child self submitted to adults who were not trustworthy. You can teach your inner child about Christ who is trustworthy and pure. As you love her and see her purity, you will become like her and be capable of guiding her to Christ. God will make His truths available to you. You must be willing to seek truth and embrace what you learn.

Adults, when they have the law, will be responsible for the light they have received. Little children are <u>always</u> blameless.

You must learn to parent your inner child and be taught by her so you can gain the blessings of eternal life. Even though the parenting and teaching of your childhood may have filled you with distortion, you can now experiment on truth. As your adult self learns then teaches, in time you will be saved whole, having gained the peace and joy promised to those who seek righteousness.

Differentiating between your adult self and your inner child. Here is a way to start to see your adult self and your inner child. The pain, guilt, and confusion you feel comes from the part of you that experienced evil. These painful experiences of being abused are felt by your inner child. You are verbalizing feelings from the inner child when you talk about how you <u>feel</u> saying, "God doesn't love me. Where was God when I was left alone?"

The way you <u>think</u> is the adult reaction to what happens in the world. You may say, "I think God is just and good to me." This is adult thinking. It is difficult to act on our thinking or beliefs, however; because most of the time we act the way we feel, not how we think.

Your inner child <u>feels</u> the first-hand experience and that is more real than any sermon or scripture. The child's understanding comes from her stage of development--she views what happened from her perspective when it happened.

If the child was taught incorrect principles and acted upon them, she did not sin. She did what someone showed or taught her to do. She was responding with all the childlike qualities God gave her.

For your adult self to become like a little child, you take the childlike qualities you already have and apply truth, after recognizing lies. When this happens, the adult self responds to God, and is able to teach the inner child to overcome distortions. By doing this you move forward to healing.

As a child you responded to the teaching of your physical care givers. Now respond to the teaching of your spiritual care giver, Heavenly Father, with the same childlike attributes you exhibited in your youth. This is an incredible lesson to learn from your inner child.

Conclusion:

1. Little children are without sin and are not accountable.

2. Inner children will be able to come to the Savior when they learn they are children of God.

3. Learn to differentiate thinking and feeling to tell if you are on an adult or child's level.

4. As you nurture your inner child, her qualities will become yours.

<u>CHAPTER SIX</u>

BEHOLDING AS IN A GLASS OF GLORY

"For if any be a hearer of the word, and not a doer, he is like unto a man beholding his natural face in a glass:
"For he beholdeth himself, and goeth his way, and straightway forgetteth what manner of man he was"
(James 1:23-24).

In order to heal you learn what God would have you do. You must bring yourself to action as you work toward the desires of your heart to be near goodness and find God's peace. You will be stuck in a cycle of pain holding you back from progression until you can see God's view by following His Spirit. You may never experience how God sees you without having loving communication with Him that moves you closer toward His merciful view.

You will learn experience by experience, line upon line, and as you do, you will still be all you were and more as you look through His glass of glory.

"But as we all, with open face beholding as in a glass the glory of the Lord, are changed into the same image from glory to glory, even as by the Spirit of the Lord" (2 Cor. 3:18).

FOLLOWING THE DIRECTION OF THE HOLY SPIRIT

Why is it so hard to recognize the Holy Spirit?

How can I tell if the voices I hear are from the Holy Spirit or from within me?

Each of us would love to have a map to guide us through our healing. It would be wonderful to have every path clearly marked, detours posted, and dangerous curves boldly labeled. We've been promised that the Holy Ghost will guide us, but how do we recognize that still small voice so we can follow the Spirit?

People who have been through abuse may have a lot of inner voices. When they hear a voice, it may be difficult to tell whether it is from within themselves or from the Holy Spirit. They feel they don't receive guidance or may not recognize it when it comes, feeling the thoughts are "crazy thinking." They may fear that if they listen to these promptings they will no longer be in control.

Because abuse controlled you, you may protect yourself from any direction which causes you to feel out of control. Protecting yourself was beneficial in the past. It kept you feeling safe and keeping yourself safe led you to become a survivor. But those actions may now hold you back from thriving in your road to wholeness.

Nov. 23, 1980. I think my <u>biggest</u> problem is prayer. I plead and beg for help and when I get the answer I know not where the answer is coming from--Satan or God. Let me tell you, Satan can really fool you. I've prayed and had both negative and positive feelings about this. Who is sending which messages?

234

When you seek the Lord He gives answers to your prayers to guide you out of your brokenness. As you follow His guidance you can put cause and effect together and learn whom you can trust.

The Spirit of God does dwell in you if you are obediently trying to do what you can to follow truth. In other words, taking a risk to act on guidance from the Spirit within will teach you about God's loving help that is available to you. Here is a pattern to follow to help you identify when the Holy Spirit is directing you.

PATTERN FOR HEALING

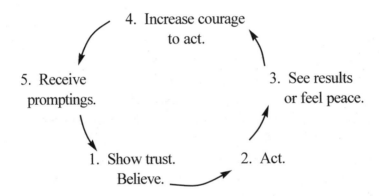

1. Learn to trust your inspiration. You do receive God's direction. Thoughts come into your mind--impressions to do things--but you may not trust yourself. You may think, *That's just me. It is just my idea. It's not a safe idea because I can't trust myself to make good decisions.*

The way to test this is to act. See what happens when you act on the idea that comes to your mind. Trust these ideas enough to test them out. If you get an idea to call a friend, think about the worst thing that could happen if you call. Follow your impressions to see what happens. What was benefited by the call? Who was helped? How?

Most of the time if you have a thought to do something positive, you are feeling divine direction. You will learn what is and isn't the spirit of the Holy Ghost as you act on the inspiration you feel. Peace should come in connection with promptings even if it only lasts briefly.

As you learn to trust God, you will become more observant about His guidance. You must tell yourself, "I don't see the outcome, but I will risk doing what I am asked." Just as you drink milk before you eat meat--you can try following impressions that are safe before you try following promptings that are a little scarier like getting out of a relationship or looking for a new therapist.

2. Act promptly. God will give you direction, but if you don't act you may lose your opportunity to receive the help. Help comes like open windows. The windows may not always be open, so timing is important. Seize the moment--act quickly to follow the spirit of truth.

Jonah was one who did not follow the direction he received. God asked Jonah to preach to the wicked people in Ninevah. Jonah didn't want to so he fled. We all know how he boarded a ship and a storm came up. Jonah was cast into the sea where he was swallowed by a great fish. Jonah prayed to God and was brought to dry land after three days. (See Jonah 1-2.)

Your consequences probably won't be as dramatic as Jonah's, but you will find if you don't follow divine guidance, you are left on your own to figure things out. (See *Depression, p.31.*)

God knows everything and will help you know what to

do. Most of the time you will not understand the end result from the beginning because you don't see what God sees. Heavenly Father sees the whole picture.

You only see the here and now and do not see clearly where your actions will lead you. You must test out trusting for God to show you He is available to direct your steps in life. When you do what God wants you to do, you are able to progress to Him.

3. Peace comes from the Holy Ghost. God will not take away your agency. He will not step in and force you to follow His guidance even though He knows you will have inner conflicts as you try. He values agency too much. Growth in happiness comes as you choose and work to act on His will.

Conflicts will come in the form of doubt and fear. Satan will place doubts in your mind telling you the feelings are not from God. He will whisper that you are hearing your own thoughts and you can't trust yourself. "After all," he'll say, "You've trusted or followed actions of others that were not right before." He might cunningly suggest that when you were abused as a child, God did not rescue you. Why would God rescue you now?

God, through the Holy Ghost, calls out to you. Then God, through the Savior, waits for you to come to Him by following the Holy Ghost's direction. The Savior is the great healer, He will heal as you follow His Spirit's direction to come to Him.

If you use your agency to follow God, you will notice an increase of strength and then an easing of your pain will follow.

Remember, peace comes when you feel the Spirit of the Holy Ghost. Satan cannot duplicate this feeling. For example, when you write in a journal, you can write down God's directions with ideas or plans of what you should do. When you look at your journal later, you will know what you have written is right because you will remember your peaceful feeling at the time you received the insight.

The Holy Spirit will work through your heart and mind to tell you what to do. There is a great advantage to this. You can receive two witnesses of what to do. The adult (or thinking self) and the child (or feeling self) can both look at what you are being guided to do. The Spirit will whisper to your heart and your mind. Two parts of yourself receive a witness--your adult and child.

4. Increase courage by overcoming fear. You may feel fearful about following inspiration, but you fear what <u>might</u> happen--the consequences. For example, you might feel fearful about going into therapy, breaking off a relationship, or chang-ing a job because you don't know what will happen after you act.

Imagine the worst case scenario. Can you live with that? The worst seldom happens. As you examine your fears, you will find many feelings originate from your inner child. Respond to the Spirit rather than letting fear bind you. Learn impressions are safe, even though the consequences which follow may be unknown.

You gain courage when you follow the Holy Ghost. God's Holy Spirit is a trustworthy friend, a peaceful com-panion, and a link to home. God is concerned about your lasting welfare and will lead you to moments that may be hard but have lasting peaceful results.

5. Do your part to receive inspiration. Matthew explains the law God follows, "Ask, and it shall be given you; seek, and ye shall find; knock, and it shall be opened unto you" (Matt. 7:7).

Many times God the Father won't intercede without you asking for help because that would take away your agency. He is waiting for you to ask. "Behold, I stand at the door, and knock: if any man hear my voice, and open the door, I will come in to him, and will sup with him, and he with me" (Rev. 3:20).

As you begin the road to following God's ways, it is through the Lord's Holy Spirit you come to Christ. God can't answer some prayers the way you ask Him to because it would interfere with someone's agency. I have prayed for people to be stopped from doing evil. God won't thwart that person's agency. (See *Feeling Abandoned by God, p. 204*.)

What God can do is strengthen you, enlighten your mind, and guide you to learn a time or a way to escape. He will help you endure to the end. He has comforted me and guided me to people who will help.

To become close to God you must learn which prayers God can answer and learn how to hear His answers. I've been told that 80% of the time you feel you have an idea from Deity and follow it, you will later see that indeed it was God's guiding hand.

Don't discount impressions. Don't decide insightful thoughts are from you. Don't discount feelings because they take you out of your comfort zone. (See *Depression, p. 31*.)

You must be willing to take a risk. Staying "comfortable" will ultimately cause depression and destructive behavior. Taking risks is spiritually safe because it will lead you to progression, peace, increasing your self esteem, and recognizing God's hand in your life.

Conclusion:

1. You can learn to recognize the Holy Ghost as you act promptly on the Spirit's truths you receive.

2. It takes faith and work to receive answers. Start with the safe direction. Work at being obedient and following the feelings of the Lord's Spirit.

3. Trust the Holy Ghost. Following the Spirit will lead to peace and progress.

4. There are consequences for not heeding the Spirit.

5. You can feel the Holy Spirit through thoughts and feelings. This will help your adult (thinking) self and your child (feeling) self.

TRUST

How is trusting God any different than trusting an authority figure who hurt me?

Why do I feel like I can never trust anyone again-- especially God?

Abuse leaves you feeling abandoned and betrayed. You have to regain trust and the only way to do that is through God. Any other way is trusting in the arm of flesh.

Many abuse victims do not trust anyone, including the Savior. They may not realize that they don't trust God because they are trying so hard to be good. They are making up for feelings of guilt rather than trusting in God.

God is trustworthy. After you have been through a lot of pain, you want the peace associated with being close to the Lord. But because He stands back and allows you to feel pain, sometimes your relationship with Jesus can feel abusive.

Your relationship with God is not going to feel totally consistent because of inner or external chaos. You won't always feel peace when you seek the Lord's hand in your life. You might not always feel the Spirit when you do what is right.

Jesus is always consistent in the fact that His motives are always for our benefit. Remember, Paul taught, "Though he were a Son, yet learned he obedience by the things which he suffered;

"And being made perfect, he became the author of eternal salvation unto all them that obey him" (Heb. 5:8-9). God is trustworthy. His acts are selfless while the abuser's acts are selfish.

As you learn how to weed out your inner voices and external expectations from God's voice, your inner child's distorted fears, pain, and confusion will ease and she can be taught to trust and follow the Spirit. When you act from your adult knowledge, you are showing trust in God and teaching your inner self to trust God. You must trust your inspiration even after the peaceful moment of direction is past and the voice of the fearful inner child is being felt. (See *Adult and Inner Child Conflict, p. 119*.)

It has been said that it is better to be trusted than to be loved. God is completely trustworthy so you are advised, "Trust in the Lord with all thine heart; and lean not unto thine own understanding.

"In all thy ways acknowledge him, and he shall direct thy paths" (Prov. 3:5-6).

You are never told to trust in man or the arm of flesh. You are to trust in God by learning to recognize the voice of God and follow the promptings He gives through the Holy Spirit.

Why Trust is Essential. When I was going through the healing process, I remember feeling I couldn't even trust myself. I would try to find answers on my own and realize I was lost.

I learned I wasn't supposed to have all the answers,

241

God would direct me to find answers. As I followed where God was directing me, I found that if I followed inspiration from God, and kept moving forward (even when I didn't know where I was headed) I would be in a better circumstance than if I had followed my own counsel. Instead of feeling determined to do things on my own, I found safety in God's guidance.

We need God. We can't progress without Him. However, we have to risk to be able to trust God. We must show trust by following His direction and living close to His will.

After being out of the country for some time, I wanted to find security at home. I decided I was going to go home and marry the young man I had been dating for several years. I tried to force or create a circumstance for this to happen.

I prayed to seek God's inspiration on what I should do when I got home. I was prompted to return to college and major in Early Childhood Development. Following God's counsel rather than forcing my own decision has given me lifelong rewards rather than lifelong regret. (See *Following the Direction of the Holy Spirit, p. 234.)*

I wasn't ready to marry and my relationship was based on a fantasy--not a good foundation for marriage. Because I followed the Spirit's guidance to go to school rather than marry right away I continued to heal so I could be successful in marriage at a later time.

My studies in Early Childhood Development built a foundation of learning that helped my adult self learn about normal childhood thinking and behavior. This set the stage for me to discover and heal my inner children. The Lord's way truly had enduring rewards.

Blessings that come from trusting God. What has God promised those who trust him?

He will direct you for good. "The Lord redeemeth the

soul of his servants: and none of them that trust in him shall be desolate" (Ps. 34:22). God is completely trustworthy. You can learn this as you accept direction from Him and wait to see the outcome. The conviction comes after you practice the principle.

You will become conquerors of your enemies. Satan is the enemy and he does not want you to trust God. He wants you to heed the fearful cries of the inner child. When you believe the distorted thinking caused from the abuse, you stay in bondage to Satan, the enemy. God is more powerful than Satan. "And the God of peace shall bruise Satan under your feet shortly. The grace of our Lord Jesus Christ be with you" (Rom.16:20).

He will deliver you from bondage. If you will turn to the Lord with full purpose of heart, and put your trust in him, and serve him with diligence, he will deliver you out of bondage.

Bondage comes from the inner child trying to heal. God will help you heal from this bondage. He wants you to have courage to follow His direction out of bondage. God does not ask you to merely live with pain. He is waiting patiently for you to choose to trust Him. He knows the path to recovery and will lead you out of your pain.

You will be delivered out of your trials. God promises when you follow His voice and do what He directs rather than that which keeps you comfortable, you will see His hand in the result. You will be miraculously led by His Hand. This deliverance will take you into life eternal following God into His kingdom.

You will be lifted up at the last day. God tests and refines His people. Your struggles can sanctify and refine you so you are worthy to live with Him.

"As many as I love, I rebuke and chasten. . .

"To him that overcometh will I grant to sit with me in my

throne, even as I also overcame, and am set down with my Father in his throne" (Rev. 3:19, 21).

You will receive immeasurable blessings as you trust God. Although you have been betrayed by others in the past, exercise a particle of faith to try to trust your Heavenly Father. Start by following promptings from the Spirit of God. You will start to see God's hand in your life leading you to Him.

Conclusion:
1. Trust is difficult because of past experiences.
2. Trust is essential because you need God's guidance in your life.
3. As you trust God, He will deliver you.

SUBMISSION
My perpetrator demanded submission. Why would God ask me to submit?
How is submission different from bondage?

It may be difficult to see that submitting to the Lord is freedom and submitting to someone else is bondage. God wants you to freely come to Him because you love Him and He loves you. He offers freedom not bondage, peace not torment, love not shame. He doesn't want you to submit to Him to bring you into bondage. He knows all and you can trust Him.

Why is submission so important? It is because you must overcome what you want and do as God asks.

"But the natural man receiveth not the things of the Spirit of God: for they are foolishness unto him: neither can he know them, because they are spiritually discerned.

"For who hath known the mind of the Lord, that he may

instruct him? But we have the mind of Christ" (1 Cor. 2:14, 16).

When you overcome the "natural man" you can learn to be instructed by God. You must learn to discern spiritual things. As you learn to follow the Holy Spirit you can become spiritually educated. The more you learn spiritually, the more you realize you can submit to a loving, all-knowing God. Indeed it is a privilege.

Submissiveness is a childlike quality you need to obtain to become a saint. Your inner child was a warrior, she submitted to someone even though he hurt her. Now teach her how to submit to God and experience His goodness. Submitting to God helps you become spiritually discerning as you take a risk to follow divine counsel. Part of overcoming the "natural man" is a willingness to submit.

Submit to God, not man. Some people blindly trust and submit to the arm of flesh. They stay in unhealthy relationships believing God wants them to stay there. God is the only one to whom you should wholly submit. You need to discover God's will for you so your trust and submission is to God, not to others.

As you learn God's will, you can make sure it matches the teachings of those you follow. If you follow teachings that are not consistent with God, you are following the will of man which will not lead you to peace and progression. Submitting is part of a pattern that prepares you to receive God's help and blessings.

God knows the way to deliver you. God will show you the path to healing if you ask for His help and receive His guidance. Don't be like the bird a friend of mine found trapped in the roof of her garage. She did all she could to help the bird.

It refused to move down to the opening and aimlessly searched for another way out. The bird refused to accept my friend's help, trust her direction, or submit to her will. It appeared to be determined to find its own deliverance.

My friend returned time and time again to see if the bird still needed help. Finally the bird accepted her guidance and left the garage, exhausted and weary. How often are you like the bird, determined to do everything your own way? Do you realize God is trying desperately to show you the way out of your pain?

Let God know you appreciate what He has done. As you submit, you will learn to trust Him and learn that He is the only true source of lasting growth and happiness. (See *Gratitude, p. 280*.)

Ways to show submission:
- Keep the commandments. (See *Second Sins, p. 171*.)
- Pray to God. (See *Prayer, p. 247*.)
- Follow the direction of the Holy Spirit. (See *Following the Direction of the Holy Spirit, p. 234*.)
- Become like a child. (See *What Does God Think of Your Inner Child? p. 215*.)

You must submit to God because He knows all. He will lead you to a far better place, a promised land within yourself. At times He will ask you to do things you don't understand, but if you follow with full purpose, you will see and understand later. You will be in awe of all God knows and has prepared for you. You will see that without Him you are nothing, but with God you can do everything.

Conclusion:
1. Submitting to God is different from submitting to anyone else.

2. Submission to God will lead you to healing and perfection.

3. You submit to Heavenly Father by being obedient and trying to be like Him.

PRAYER

Why do I need to pray?
God wasn't there for me during the abuse, why would He be there now?

There are many reasons why abuse victims may find it hard to pray. They are confused about or angry with God because they feel like He abandoned them as a child so they see no reason to communicate with Him and try to develop a relationship now. They may doubt God's existence. They have never seen Him, how do they know He really exists?

Other victims have a deep faith in God, but struggle with submitting to anyone--heavenly though God may be. The thought of kneeling in prayer is uncomfortable. (See *Kneeling Sabotages My Heartfelt Prayer, p. 253.*)

Nov. 6, 1994. I have a very heavy weakness, a weakness grievous to me. I have not had constant, sincere, soul-searching prayers for years. I don't understand why it has been such a difficult challenge for me, but I would like to explore this on paper and try to discover how to over-come this.

The first thing that comes to mind is that being close to God involves an emotional closeness. If a person is not open emotionally, it is difficult to be close to anyone. Actually, it is impossible. I believe the reason has a lot to do with trust and feeling secure. It also has to do with my

*willingness to feel pain. After so much numbness, holding it
in is safer than expressing pain that is stuffed deep and may
be more overwhelmingly explosive than I know how to
handle.*

*I also wonder if my weakness in not praying is
Satan's ploy to stop me from growth, progression and
truth. He tells me information that is false and I believe it.*

*I have so many areas I want to grow in and it is up
to me to overcome my weaknesses so I can. This week I
have two goals: 1. Pray three times a day sincerely. The
other goals are not to even be recognized until I pray. 2. I
will study about trusting God, Satan's plot to stop prayer,
and frequency in prayer. I'm sure there are other topics
that I'll study, but maybe as I strive to learn about closeness with God, my heart will pour out in closeness to Him.*

God is the author of your healing. Without the help
of God you are left to yourself to figure out how to heal. Once
you learn that God is not only an ally, but the author of your
healing process, you realize that without Him you have nothing.
With Him you have hope for true and lasting peace or
deliverance. (See *Trust, p. 240.*)

Prayer is not a religious formality or a tradition. It
literally is how to become close to God. "The Lord is far from
the wicked: but he heareth the prayer of the righteous" (Prov.
15:29).

You can gain incredible insight when you pray and take
time to ponder. You can learn what God might tell you if He
were here in person. I believe we communicated with God and
felt His love before we came to earth. Our time spent being
near Him in this life rekindles our memory of who He is and
who we are.

When my heart aches and I search for direction and

answers, there are many people to whom I can go. They may offer advice. They may give blank looks saying, "I wish I understood." Most people have good intentions, but they cannot do what God can do.

God hears us, understands the words we can't say, and will reassure our heart. Only God, through His Spirit, knows how to tap into our heart and mind. He is the one that leads us out of bondage. "Whosoever shall call on the name of the Lord shall be delivered" (Joel 2:32).

Find ways to remove barriers between you and God. Choosing to be unbelieving or to stay angry with God is choosing to go through this world of sorrow alone--without a lasting refuge, without true hope. Satan wants you to feel alone. You are most vulnerable when you believe Satan's words and follow his paths which lead to more pain, more loneliness, and life without knowing the one who holds the eternal light you need.

When I attended church as a child I learned a song about God's love. I always enjoyed this song and it strengthened me. A survivor of abuse told me that to her it was the most painful song in her church experience. If God was telling her that he sent her to "parents kind and dear" as the song said, and those parents neglected and abused her, then what kind of God was He?

I was amazed because I had never struggled with that part of the song. As I hummed the words to myself, I realized what I had done in my pain. I remedied the song to fit my need and sang the words, "parents *kind of dear*." I suppose any parent, even an abuser is "kind of dear" at times. I don't see myself as completely "kind and dear" as I stumble through parenting, but I can be "kind of dear" without much failure.

Seek ways to remedy the little things that cause a

barrier between you and God so that you can feel His love. A loving Father in Heaven is there for you. He wants you to come to Him so He can lead you back to your heavenly home. As you try to go to Him in prayer, He will literally lead, guide, and walk beside you. He will teach you what you must know to live with Him someday.

Conclusion:

1. Many abuse victims have a difficult time with prayer because of anger or unbelief.

2. When you choose unbelief, you choose to try to heal without God, the author of your healing.

3. Prayer is the way you become close to God.

FEELING VICTIMIZED IN PRAYER

God wasn't there for me during the abuse; how do I know God isn't an ally with the perpetrator?

If God wants me to submit to Him, how is He different from Satan or the perpetrator who both want my submission?

After abuse a lot of relationships feel confrontational. An abuse victim finds it very difficult to confront or submit. She feels victimized to formally express needs, wants, and desires. She wants God and others to know what she needs so they can rescue her, but she doesn't want to beg for her needs. It is very difficult to express the need to be released from her trauma.

For me it was a confrontation to pray on my knees, but natural to pray continually in my heart. Every minute was difficult and only the silent cry felt safe. Most abused children learn to say their first sincere prayers in silence. It is also the only safe way to pray because no one can hear them and hurt them again because of reactions to their prayer. (See *Kneeling Sabotages My Heartfelt Prayer, p. 253.*)

When you pray, even when you are not on your knees, you feel like you are submitting to another's desires and those desires may be painful for you. God requests, "Submit yourselves therefore to God. Resist the devil, and he will flee from you" (James 4:7).

Submission to anyone makes you feel like a victim. You may feel like you are trying to stand up to the perpetrator, begging for him to give you something. It makes me feel sick to remember the feeling. (See *Submission, p. 244.*)

God is different from Satan or a perpetrator. God asks us to do difficult things. The perpetrator also wants or asks us to do difficult things. There are differences, of course. God's difficult requests help us grow. The perpetrator has no blessing for us. His requests are selfish--they are only for his benefit. This outline shows the difference between God, Satan, and the perpetrator.

Satan	**God**	**Perpetrator**
Hates agency	Gives agency	Abuses agency
Distorts truth	Offers truth	Hates truth
Wants us in eternal misery and bondage	Wants us to have lasting joy and progression	Cares nothing for our well being
		Cares only for himself

Based on her development, the inner child sees similarities between God and Satan, or God and the perpetrator. She has no ability to see intricate and abstract detail. As an adult you can comprehend that God is asking you to do hard things within your ability and only for your gain. The inner child does not understand this.

Prayer is the most ideal way to release the pain, but for some it is too hard to share the pain with God. Your inner child may feel God caused the pain. To seemingly share pain with "an enemy" may confuse your inner child and be too difficult.

Don't feel guilty for feeling this way. God understands this, too. This does not mean you are evil. It means your inner child doesn't recognize the perpetrator. She doesn't understand who really caused the pain and why the pain was allowed.

God understands what you cannot understand.
Our 14-month-old son sucked a hydrocarbon (cleaning fluid) into his lungs one night. He was sitting right next to me. I saw him holding the bottle and cried, "No, Jamin!" He sucked it into his lungs while looking into my eyes.

There was shock in his eyes. Pain and disbelief that came over his face. We did what we could. We ran him to the emergency room. Nurses and doctors put tubes down him, needles in him, an inhalator down him to help him breathe.

All I could do was stand back and watch. I could do nothing more. I could pray for him, but as far as he was concerned I had caused his pain. He thought I was the one who was allowing all this to happen. I was the enemy. This was baffling to him.

There was no way for me to show Jamin that what I was doing was the best I could for him. I was standing back because I loved him. I wanted him to live. I wanted him to be able to come home with me again. I knew no other way to allow for him to heal and I knew he probably would not understand. In fact there was no way at 14 months for him to comprehend the things I knew as a mother.

Your Father in Heaven, too, loves you very much. Your inner child does not understand what Heavenly Father knows. God does not expect your inner child to understand

252

any more than I expected my baby boy to understand. But your adult self can teach your inner child that it was out of deep love for you that God stood back so you could live and somehow come home to Him again.

As you follow promptings to pray, you can teach your inner child that God is the only one who can never be a perpetrator. He is the deliverer, your greatest ally. As you keep praying and show your inner child patterns of simple prayers answered, your inner child will eventually see God as a friend, a parent, a nurturer of the soul.

Submission is difficult. God is the only safe person to whom you can submit because He will never take advantage of you or hurt you. He is the one person you can safely trust.

If you trust God a little at a time you will be able to internalize the potential of your relationship with Him. You will learn that God sees beyond what you know or see here on earth. He will guide you to that which you are truly seeking and cannot find on your own.

Conclusion:

1. Prayer can feel confrontational as you ask God to bless you and meet your needs.

2. Teach your inner child about God's goodness and trustworthiness. Teach her how God is different than Satan and a perpetrator.

KNEELING SABOTAGES MY HEARTFELT PRAYER

Why do I struggle to kneel in prayer?
Will God hear my prayer if I pray in my heart?

Many abuse victims suffer with the inability to pray on their knees. Praying on one's knees can bring a feeling of

253

submission much like a victim felt during her abuse, causing her to feel victimized again. Kneeling may have been part of the abuse, but mostly being on one's knees brings a feeling of inappropriate submission.

When you feel victimized by God you have a distorted view of the Lord's will. You may think God feels you deserve to be in pain. You need to see Heavenly Father in a whole new way. Prayer should be a refuge, a safe place. When you force prayer on your knees, you may feel like an enemy is with you. God does not want you to feel victimized.

Purposes of kneeling in prayer. I believe kneeling is meant to bring a feeling of reverence for God. Kneeling is a way to show respect and honor. If the act of kneeling ostracizes you from God, it defeats its purpose and sabotages you from gaining the trust, closeness and all the blessings that are meant to be gained from communicating with God.

I set a goal to pray on my knees because I knew power comes from praying on knees rather than praying in one's heart. I have felt tremendous love from Heavenly Father when I prayed on my knees because I wanted to, rather than because I felt obligated to. Some people, however, can't get past the anxiety from praying on their knees until they heal completely.

I struggled with formal prayer and had to explore how to solve the problem because of my desire to draw closer to God through obedience to pray formally to Him.

May 24, 1992. When I have personal prayers, I must speak verbally. If I pray in my mind only I feel tired and my mind wanders. I also do not feel what I am thinking very poignantly. Because of this I need to change what I am doing--to kneel up straight and to speak out loud so that I am more in tune with what I am doing.

How do you pray until you can kneel? Pray for a change of heart about prayer, then pray in your heart until you can pray on your knees. It may not work to pray on your knees until you are ready. Pray in your heart until you can come to your knees feeling peace rather than feeling victimized. There are many scriptures that command us to pray continually, only a few suggest praying on our knees.

While watching a movie, my daughter, Katilyn, and I were focused as the actors struggled with a problem. Katilyn asked, "Mommy, why don't they just pray about it?"

I thought, *They're not on their knees--that's what she sees. But how can we tell they are not fervently praying?* Fervent prayer needn't always be on one's knees.

Will God answer your silent prayers? You are valuable to your Heavenly Father. God will answer your prayers and deliver you from bondage. If your prayer is from the heart instead of from your knees, God will still hear it.

Hannah could not bear a child and "in bitterness of soul" she "prayed unto the Lord and wept sore" (1 Sam. 1:10).

"And it came to pass, as she continued praying before the Lord, that Eli [the priest] marked [or saw] her mouth.

"Now Hannah, she spake in her heart; only her lips moved, but her voice was not heard" (v. 12-13).

When questioned, Hannah told the priest, "I am a woman of a sorrowful spirit: I . . . have poured out my soul before the Lord" (v.15).

Then Eli answered and said, "Go in peace: and the God of Israel grant thee thy petition that thou hast asked of him" (v.17). So the woman went her way, "and the Lord remembered her . . . She bare a son, and called his name Samuel" (v. 20).

Later Hannah said to the priest, "O my Lord, as thy soul liveth, my lord, I am the woman that stood by thee here, praying unto the Lord" (v. 26).

"For this child I prayed; and the Lord hath given me my petition which I asked of him" (v. 27). Hannah then sang praises to the Lord. Through her silent prayers Hannah received the wish of her heart.

How does God deliver people from bondage? You can learn much about bondage and deliverance from Moses and his people. Notice, God didn't deliver them all at once. He made them stronger so they could carry their burdens. This can happen for you, too. Watch for little ways you are made stronger to carry your burdens. As you submit with patience and cheerfulness, God will also deliver you. (See *Deliverance is a Process, p. 63.*)

You can begin to do this by expressing gratitude to the Lord each time you realize He has helped you. Hannah did this as she sang praises to the Lord (see 1 Sam. 2:1). In this way you witness to God that you recognize His hand in your life, then you will feel an increase of love and trust towards God during prayers. Showing gratitude is a bonding part of prayer, a key to increasing the feelings and impressions you receive from the Lord. (See *Praying with Gratitude and Real Intent, p. 283.*)

You can pray in all sorts of places and circumstances. Even when you are not formally praying, you can have a prayer in your heart for your welfare and the welfare of others.

You may feel your abuse has put you in a bondage as literal as the bondage Moses and his people experienced. Your deliverance will come the same way, through a comforting Savior who will ease your burdens as you go to Him in prayer. Start by praying in your heart and as you heal you will eventually long or desire to pray on your knees.

Conclusion:
1. You may need to pray in your heart until you

can pray on your knees.

    2. God will hear the prayers from your heart.

    3. Your heartfelt prayers will lead you out of bondage.

FORTIFYING YOURSELF WITH GOD'S ARMOR

What is "the armor of God"?
How will "the armor of God" protect me?

When you put on "the armor of God," you are strengthened to do the good you long to do. You are also protected from evils that destroy and falsehoods that cause detours.

    David, of the Old Testament, was a boy who trusted in God and used the Lord's protection. He armed himself with God's armor. One of Saul's servants described David as a "mighty valiant man, and a man of war, and prudent in matters, and a comely person, and the Lord is with him" (1 Sam. 16:18).

    What did David do to form his character with virtues that caused others to look so highly on a young boy?

Faith in God's power. First, David was a shepherd who had faith in God's deliverance. He acknowledged God's protection in his life telling Saul, "The Lord. delivered me out of the paw of the lion and out of the paw of the bear" (1 Sam. 17:37).

    David had faith that God's protection would continue to bless him. When Saul tried to dissuade David from facing Goliath because David was "but a youth" (v. 33), David replied, "The Lord that delivered me out of the paw of the lion, and out of the paw of the bear, he will deliver me out of the hand of this Philistine" (v. 37).

    You can gain faith in God the same way David did.

Look for times God has blessed you or protected you. Acknowledge the Lord's hand in your life. Face new challenges with the confidence--or hope--that God will again bless and protect you.

Protection in the strength of God. Second, David refused to be armed in strange attire. When the time came for David to battle against the Philistine, Goliath, Saul attempted to dress David for battle. "And Saul armed David with his armour, and he put an helmet of brass upon his head; also he armed him with a coat of mail" (1 Sam. 17:38).

David hesitated to go to battle dressed in Saul's armor. "And David said to Saul, I cannot go with these; for I have not proved them. And David put them off him" (v. 39). David knew God was his strength. Saul's protective armor was not what he needed. He needed to depend on God.

When friends, neighbors, and therapists try to arm you with worldly philosophies, realize they want to help you just as Saul wanted to help David. Try their ideas on for size, but before you use them compare them with God's truths. If the new ideas feel compatible with God's truths, they will probably provide comfort and protection. You can feel safe in using them.

Hold to known truths as you move into unknown experiences. Third, David clung to truths he knew from past successes and trusted them to hold true. He had fought battles against the enemy (the lion and bear) in his field of sheep. As he prepared to fight Goliath he chose the same weapons.

"And he took his staff in his hand, and chose him five smooth stones out of the brook, and put them in a shepherd's bag which he had, even in a scrip; and his sling was in his hand: and he drew near to the Philistine" (v. 40).

What are your "weapons?" What has been successful for you in the past? Do you find strength in prayer? Do you know how to listen for the Holy Spirit? Have you learned how to surround yourself with good, uplifting companions? Use the positive things that have worked in the past to build on what you will do in the future.

In battles, stand strong to the end. We all know David was successful in choosing to battle in the strength of the Lord. "So David prevailed over the Philistine with a sling and with a stone, and smote the Philistine, and slew him; but there was no sword in the hand of David" (v. 50). David had opposition before he fought Goliath. His brothers did not support him. The king, an authority figure, tried to change David's way of fighting--for his own good.

It is imperative in your fight to heal that you hang onto those things you learn are true. David conquered the enemy the Lord's way, not the popular way. Some will not support you. Some will try to get you to change. Learn step-by-step what God would have you do, then stick with Him to the end, don't give up, and you will prevail.

God's armor is internal. This section is all about armor. To look at David, observers would say he did not wear armor. What did David wear? He wore the armor of God. In Ephesians we read, "Put on the whole armour of God, that ye may be able to stand against the wiles of the devil" (Eph. 6:11).

Imagine, God's armor can even protect you against your greatest enemy--Satan. You need not be deceived by his inaccurate and damaging philosophies. When you hear his taunts saying, "You will never heal" or "You are unworthy for God's help" you can stand up to those falsehoods. You can heal. You are worthy of God's help.

The armor of God protects all of your most vulnerable spiritual areas. Your "loins girt about with truth, and having on the breastplate of righteousness" (v. 14). Your "feet [are] shod with the preparation of the gospel of peace" (v. 15).

You carry a shield of faith which shield enables you "to quench all the fiery darts of the wicked" (v. 16). Then you take "the helmet of salvation, and the sword of the Spirit, which is the word of God" (v. 17). You do this as you pray always and implement the Spirit, persevering to sainthood.

You can implement God's internal shields to guard your life from the evil influences of the world when you have faith in God, when you refuse to accept ideas that are not of the Lord, when you hold to God's way, and when you endure to the end of your battle. As you work with your inner child, remember to this end do you fight--that it may be said of you, "the Lord is with us" (1 Sam. 16:18).

Conclusion:
1. You wear God's armor when you follow His truths.
2. Evaluate philosophies of the world against God's truth to safely make decisions.
3. God's armor will protect you against Satan and his falsehoods.

STRENGTHENING AGAINST DAMAGING CYCLES

Why do I struggle with the same problems over and over again?

Why do I seem to go through the same cycles when I'm trying to overcome a problem?

If you double and triple the panes of glass in your home, you provide greater protection for it. Panes of glass joined together can provide a way to strengthen weak areas and are a type of fortification.

Fortifying is temporary, a way to protect yourself while you go to your inner child to heal, or in other words, rebuild your foundation. This strengthening will last only if you work and accomplish healing. Glass that is exposed to continual pressure day after day will eventually break. You can only free yourself from pain and damaging cycles by healing. As long as pain from trauma remains, destructive cycles will happen on hazardous, stormy days.

As you work on healing, you will go through patterns of painful coping behavior. You must strengthen yourself from weaknesses and these cycles of self-defeating practices. (See *Second Sins, p. 171; Fortifying Yourself with God's Armor, p. 257.*)

A typical cycle:

1. <u>Stop abusive behavior.</u> You are so fed up, you stop destructive or non-productive behavior. You can't stand the negative consequences of unwanted behavior.

2. <u>Feel angry at yourself.</u> You realize the impact of the negative actions and you feel angry. You inflict self punishment by saying things like, "I must be a horrible person to have done that. I must be weak and selfish." These are not healthy feelings of guilt for wrong doing that enable you to repent. These thoughts are destructive. They break you down and can cause you to feel helpless to know how to act differently.

3. <u>Refrain from the act.</u> You refrain from doing the behavior because of your self hate. You say, "I'll never do that again." Even though you are starting to feel weak, you resist succumbing to the temptation saying you are not going near it.

4. <u>Motivated to overcome bad habit.</u> Because you

have stopped for a short while and have resisted the temptation, you feel encouraged and proud of yourself. You say, "I can overcome this. I'm not so bad. I can be strong and achieve my goal. It is not so hard."

5. <u>The glass breaks.</u> You feel depression, self doubt, vulnerable. You start to feel greater temptations and weakness toward the destructive behavior, but this time you doubt yourself and do not feel strong. You feel helpless to refrain from the act. Even though you desire to resist, you feel you barely escape doing it.

It is important to note that when you feel vulnerable (like delicate glass), you are feeling the effects of abuse. You are experiencing the feelings and thought patterns of the inner child. The darkness caused by the abuse is triggered and surfaces to heal. Your temptation to start unwanted behavior is a way to control the confusion, and anxiety you feel. It is an effort to gain control over something uncontrollable.

When you return to the destructive behavior you feel a release. You may believe you will feel safer and more in control. For a short while the destructive behavior masks what you are feeling from the inner child. Soon your feelings of being trapped by the negative consequences and feelings of guilt from going against your adult self will surface. You have broken the glass meant to protect you.

6. <u>Start self-destructive behavior again.</u> Broken glass exposes you to evil. When weakened again with opposition, you are unable to clearly see how to resist the temptation. Succumbing seems the only thing to do. You feel trapped, destined, confused and without courage to resist or follow your good desires. You don't know how to overcome, and just resisting the temptation is not good enough.

In order to stop this cycle, you must add a pane of glass within yourself at step number four, where you are motivated to stop destructive behavior. While life is calm, prepare to be strong. Be prepared for times of weakness. Don't think, *I've overcome this problem so I won't worry about it any more.* Instead think, *I __will__ be tempted again if I do not prepare myself to stay away from unwanted behavior.* (See *How Do I Strengthen Myself? p. 265.*)

A scenario. For clarity, here is a typical scenario that follows a woman through the six steps:

The woman is taking medication beyond what is prescribed. She is out of commission for a few days leaving her children to fend for themselves. She neglects her obligations. She can't stand being unable to function any longer so she stops taking the drugs (step #1).

She realizes she didn't care for her children or accomplish anything while she was overdosing on the medication. She hates herself for being a bad mother and is worried what others will think of her (step #2).

She tells herself she won't overdose again. She stays away from drugs so she can be a good mother. What she really wants is for other people to believe she is a good mother (step #3).

She has good days with her children. She is back doing things that she feels others expect. She doesn't think about taking the drugs very often. She is proud of herself for doing what is "healthy." She wants to continue to be a good mother and please others such as her husband, her neighbors, and church members (step #4).

One morning the woman feels anxious and overwhelmed by her many tasks. She has many feelings at once. She can't think straight or act productively. She begins to feel like a failure in caring for her family and others. She is unable to do what she thinks others expect of her. She tells herself this will pass. She resists taking the drugs. She assures herself that things will become better. She thinks God is testing her or Satan is tempting her. She thinks, *If I hold on, I'll overcome* (step #5).

For several days she fights feelings of anxiety and inability to cope. One day it becomes even worse. She feels great anxiety, deep depression. She doesn't know where to turn or how to get out of despair. She feels she is being punished by God for being bad. She feels rejected and abandoned by others because she is a nobody if she isn't perfect. (See *Perfectionism, p. 27.*)

She feels she can't rise above her problem. She has no one to care about her, no one to help, nowhere to go. She takes drugs to dull the pain. Drugs helped her before to function without this pain. Maybe it will help if she just takes a little of what the doctor gave her. She rationalizes that the doctor gave it to her to help her (step #6). The cycle completes and starts over.

To get out of destructive cycles, you must double and triple pane weak areas. You can stop these destructive cycles if you strengthen yourself when you feel strong and capable. This will help you resist temptation when you are more vulnerable.

Conclusion:

1. Although you go through cycles of self-defeating behavior, you can strengthen yourself to stop the cycle.

2. Satan will try to break you when and where you are weak and vulnerable.

3. You can best resist Satan's destruction if you strengthen yourself and prepare for his attacks during the times

when you feel strong.

HOW DO I STRENGTHEN MYSELF?
How can I set limits?
What are some typical weak areas that need fortification?

It is important to realize that fortifications are temporary. Military leaders do not expect fortifications to win the battle for them. They are built so people are not easy prey. Fortifications help defend people against their enemy.

Your inner child is your warrior. You need to become an ally with her. She is the one that will win the battle with your adult self's guidance. It is important to fortify yourself against destructive habits so that when you and the inner child are fighting the painful battle of overcoming the effects of abuse, you can still cope with everyday life.

Weak places need fortification. Look honestly at yourself to see if any of these issues are weaknesses created by your abuse.

Abusive sexual relationships. You allow abusive sexual behavior in a relationship. You are in a sexual relation that feels abusive. You are in a relationship that feels painful physically, mentally, or emotionally. This might be in or out of marriage.

Problems with limits in sexuality. You allow more to happen physically than you want. You feel like you set boundaries and go past them. Or you are committed to a relationship, but won't have sex or can't allow sexual behavior. (See *Sexual Boundaries, p. 180; Sexuality in Marriage, p. 188.*)

Oct. 3, 1981. I have had a lot of thoughtful moments in the last few days. I am very confused about a lot of things. My biggest problem is the fact I am a flirt and I don't know how to not flirt. But even a bigger problem is the way guys react to my flirtations. They seem to take it as a very big pass . When I get alone with one of these young men, they seem to expect a little more out of me than I'm interested in giving. I want to be a morally clean girl. So what shall I do? I have to search in my heart to find the answer.

<u>Misuse of food, alcohol, prescription or hard drugs.</u> You take drugs or alcohol to cover confusion, low self-worth, inability to cope, or anger. Drugs help you mask feelings and emotions. You take drugs to escape your life because you don't know how to face it. You don't know how to cope with life without taking alcohol or drugs. You use food as a drug and overuse it or deprive yourself of it. (See *Second Sins, p. 171.*)

July 30, 1980. I want to write something that I've wanted to write for a long time. I weigh 120 pounds. I am 5'4". I hate weighing so much. I've never weighed so much before in my life so I'm going to lose weight.
My eating schedule will be:
Thursday–nothing but water.
Friday only something little for just before the parade.
Saturday will be the same.
Sunday–nothing.
Monday–a little of something at lunch.
Tuesday is my birthday and I hope I will have lost a lot of weight.
I can't stand myself. I'm just not happy with my

looks so I have to lose weight so I can regain confidence.

Abuse to yourself or others. You are sexually controlling, verbally or physically abusive. You are abusive to your body. You feel anger at yourself for your actions and can't stop.

Strengthen yourself to overcome these weak areas. Part of being strengthened or fortified while you heal is seeking the best kind of help. Don't expect yourself to break patterns on your own. Seek help from family, friends, and therapists. Find allies who will help you fortify yourself. (See *Following the Direction of the Holy Spirit, p. 234.*)

What will you do when you are vulnerable? Make a plan. When you are in the depression or self-doubt stage, it is a difficult time to find and accept help. These suggestions are not how to overcome the whole cycle permanently, this is to keep you out of the "attack or abusive stage." (See *Strengthening against Damaging Cycles, p. 260.*)

What you do after you ask for help from an outsider is very important to heal the cycle permanently. First seek the inner child and find help to heal issues that are surfacing. This action will help you work through the pain rather than burying it by taking drugs. You will realize you take drugs to dull the pain because you feel helpless. (See *Depression, p. 31.*)

How Do You Fortify Yourself?
Seek a good environment to heal. Risk a change in your surroundings. You may need to move, find new friends, or break off a relationship.

Don't beat yourself up for being vulnerable. Recognize you are vulnerable. Destructive actions like hurting yourself and others are not okay and you must take responsibility to overcome them. You may have developed these actions to survive the effects of abuse and they are no longer helpful. You can heal now, not merely get by.

Ask for help. If you are hurting others--be honest with your family about your limits. Ask for their support to have time outs, someone to call, a place to go to fortify yourself. If your eating habits are extreme, tell a friend your trial, your desires to be healthy, your need for her help. If you starve or binge food have her help you with a plan. Find ways to get support from someone to help you follow through and make a plan to abstain from destructive behavior. Seek a supportive friend that you can talk to. (See *Receiving Help from Others, p. 143; Second Sins, p.171.*)

Seek counseling. Look at your patterns of behavior together. (See *Should I Go to Therapy? p. 77.*)

Ask others to support you through prayer.

Write in your journal. See if you can recognize patterns to show when you are feeling more anxious or overwhelmed. As you write, decide what you will do now to help you focus on good and turn away from the unwanted behavior. (See *Journal Writing. p. 271.*)

Take healthy time outs when you feel stress. Release energy in a healthy environment. Exercise, read, listen to soothing music, take a hot bath, walk through a park, go to the mountains. Seek outside help with children and responsibilities while you do this.

Experiment with receiving answers to prayers and following the direction of the Holy Spirit. (See *Following the*

Direction of the Holy Spirit, p. 234.)

<u>Discover your inner child.</u> Work to connect feelings with past experience. (See *Parenting the Inner Child, p. 123.*)

<u>Study the scriptures and good books.</u> Experiment with discovering new ways to internalize and apply truth. Seek to learn truth from a new perspective--the perspective of the innocent inner child.

<u>Pray.</u> Find a safe place, a safe person, a peaceful way to let the pain out. Prayer is probably the most direct and effective way. Share your anger, fears, confusion, feelings of betrayal with God. Christ has felt all the same feelings you feel. He lived a mortal existence. He knows that life's experiences are painful. I have felt great empathy from God as I have poured out my heart to Him. (See *Prayer, p. 247.*)

Don't worry if you can't express your pain to God. Find a friend or a therapist, a safe supportive person and express your feelings about Heavenly Father and your confusion about Him. This will help you to sort out your inner pain and in time you will be able to progress from talking to a friend to talking with God.

Remember God wants to hear from you, even your words of feeling betrayed and confused, your anger and even hate. Don't be afraid to let out your feelings. It will bring incredible relief and will help you begin to feel easing of pain and sustaining from God.

Expressing pain is not the same as cursing God. It is an honest way of communicating and openly expressing what you feel. This is good.

A personal example. When I was working through some pain, I remember going in our fenced-in back yard and

269

dumping my anger and confusion on God. Where was He?
Had I done something wrong before I was born to deserve
this? Did I have so little worth to God that He should allow this
to happen to me?

What kind of God was He anyway to let so much
happen to a baby, a child? Did God call this belonging to
Him?!? As my anger and pain poured out of me, I was able to
see deeper things and begin to feel His love. I felt His Spirit as
though He was saying, "Peace to you, my daughter. I <u>do</u> love
you. I know what happened. Remember my Son who suffered
all. He suffered for you. You are worth that much."

Because I tried to communicate with God, I felt I began
a <u>real</u> coming unto God and a true rebirth in His Son's Atonement. Healing comes more directly and powerfully when you
go to the source, the one who is acquainted with all pain.

Fortification is a chance to fight the war and win. God
is your ally. Use your greatest strength. When you strengthen
yourself to fortify the weak places caused by your childhood
battle, you will be able to break damaging patterns that keep
you enslaved. As you strengthen yourself and then work on
healing your inner child through therapy, you will be able to fight
everyday battles successfully.

Conclusion:
1. Problems with morality, drugs, alcohol, abusive
behavior are typical areas that need to be fortified.
2. Find safe ways to release your pain which will fortify
you and help you heal.

JOURNAL WRITING

Why do I want to write the garbage I'm feeling?
Won't writing my feelings on paper make me feel
even more despair?

Writing in a journal is an effective way to analyze your life. Journals enable you to sort out thoughts, ideas and inspiration on paper. When you write, you see life more clearly and gain insight as to directions you should take.

Journal writing gave me power because it moved the chaos inside of me into tangible material with which I could work. It helped make my inner world and thoughts more real. I was able to make my experiences concrete again.

For journal writing to be effective, you must be honest with yourself. As you write in your journal, you will discover how you really feel about God, other people, and personal issues. Face what you really think. As you discover your true feelings, you will discover where you really are.

Sept. 5, 1984. In a few pages I will be finished with this journal. There is so much in here--trials, triumphs, joy, pain, sorrow, peace and a lot of patience and long suffering. I feel my Heavenly Father's lesson for me in my life is patience.

My journals mean a lot to me. I find there are times I can't stand to not write. I have to express myself and tell of my experiences before I can keep going. Sometimes it feels like my release. I am able to stand back and look at my life from a different point of view and see my problems and situations more clearly.

Journal writing helps change destructive or unprogressive behavior. As you discover these patterns, a

written commitment to change will give you strength to overcome. When your resolve weakens, you can refer back to the
commitment in your journal and start working on your goal
again. (See *How Do I Strengthen Myself? p. 265.*)

Experiences are like matter. Matter is neither created,
nor destroyed. It simply changes form. In the same way, your
experiences continue to exist, but your perceptions about them
may change. To compare, you can take a piece of wood and
burn it. The matter or wood still exists. It may now be ashes
and smoke, but the matter did not disappear. It still is something. Your experiences, like matter, exist after they happen.
They are held in your memory.

Wood, after it is burned, seems useless. But the ashes
can be used in fertilizer, soap, or potting soil. The wood is not
useless. It can be used for something new. In a similar way
journal writing brings the abuse experiences, thoughts, pain, and
confusion out of the abstract and into a tangible workable state
so you can do something with them. You can change the
original experience into something that will help you progress
and not hold you back. Help the inner child make the
experience tangible so you can work with it. Write down
feelings and thoughts so the experience can be examined.

As you write thoughts down, analyze your feelings.
You might say, "I've been depressed because. . ." Examine the
causes for your depression, then move to action. Write what
you plan to do to overcome the depression.

Journal writing will help you recognize and deal with
your pain. Take the pain and allow the experience to go
through you. Accept what you can carry and let the Savior
take the rest.

Journal writing will help you progress. As you write
in your journal, don't stay stuck in the pain. Write what you

want to do and how you want to progress. Set goals in your journal. Here are a few ways to use your journal to move to hope, growth, and action:

Write about the pain you feel. Analyze what may have caused the pain. Write about the problems your face.

October 9, 1990. Yesterday I talked to a counselor after freaking out for a while, and she told me to write in my journal and spend an hour a day on personal therapy. It is important that I do this because if I don't fears, doubts and pain begin to build up inside of me and I can't concentrate or deal with the world around me. I find I just am completely absorbed in myself and unaware of others. For myself and the people I deal with (school, friends, Brian, and my roommates) I must work through this daily so I can release anxiety and continue with daily life.

Brian is the most positive and yet most stressful and frightening subject in my life right now. He is wonderful to me and for me. It is almost unbelievable that someone could be so good for me and be so interested in me and I in him. How blessed can a person get? My fears toward all of this deals with my belief in myself, my trust towards the world, the unknown, and fear of a replay of my past in my life or my child's life.

Write about your gratitude. We are promised opposition in all things. Look for any evidence of good that opposes the bad in your life.

Nov. 23, 1990. I've got a lot to do to get my life in order and I'm going to take one thing at a time, implement it and when it's a habit implement a new habit. I've let

*myself believe that because I am struggling through
therapy I can be self-centered and let go of all the good
goals I had. This is wrong. I'm not happy feeling sorry for
myself and I'm not healing concentrating on myself so
much.*

*I'm going to write ten things a day that I am
specifically grateful for. My goal is to write 500. I feel I
can feel closer to God by doing this.*

   1. Good health.
   2. Peace.
   3. Car that runs.
   *4. Mom's service--perming my hair, feeding me,
doing my laundry while I was there researching my abuse.*
   5. Clean clothes.
   6. Songs of worship.
   7. Fixed neck--chiropractor.
   8. Homework.
   9. Scriptures.
   10. Family.

<u>List strengths</u> you have that will help you heal and
overcome your pain.

*Nov. 29, 1986. Here are some of my strengths: I
am good at organizing things. I like to organize work and
parties and my life. I love the feeling of being organized.*

*I am good at showing people I love them. I love all
kinds of people and I love expressing those feelings through
service and a good hug now and then. I love buying gifts
for others.*

*I am good at understanding people. I understand
their feelings when they express their trials.*

I enjoy singing. I can touch people when I sing and

I feel the words.

I have a love for God that helps me to stay close to Him and feel His influence.

I love children. I have patience. I am very patient with other people and in difficult situations.

I am childlike. I see the world through childlike eyes. I know what is in the world as far as evil, but I like to look for and magnify the good and warmth. I believe I can be who I want. I do not have to absorb what is around me.

I am determined. I will accomplish goals. I will overcome obstacles and trials and problems. I am determined to continue to become a better person in my eyes. I am determined to achieve my life-long goals and I will not give up.

I know right from wrong. I know what I should do to continue to progress. I know what God wants me to do and I know I am on the proper road to get there. I want to be a good example, and most times I am.

I can do anything I set my mind to. I am good at enduring well. Sometimes the problems stop me from seeing clearly, but I endure it well and I try to help others and do the best I can with what I've got.

I have great potential and as I go through a trial I see a better me, a stronger, more understanding me. I am closer to my potential. I like myself. I am a good person. I am not a showy person and others might not see a lot of my strengths, but I've got a lot of good.

Write goals. Write specifically how and why you will accomplish the goals. Set a target date to achieve the goal. Express gratitude for the resources you have to accomplish your goals. I wrote these goals the summer I graduated from high school.

July 21, 1982. I've decided I want to work on growing spiritually. I need to make a list of qualities and abilities I would like to possess in the future. I want to think big--think in terms of eternity. So I've decided that I would write down some of my very special desires to obtain in the future. These are dreams, but I think they--in a sense--can be goals and can be achieved also.

I would like to be a speaker for young people and adults.

I would someday like to write a book about some-thing pertaining to the gospel.

I would like to become a sewer of clothing.

I would like to sing when asked, beautifully and well balanced, but most of all touching the hearts of those who can hear and understand.

I would like to marry and not think of that as the end, but only the beginning of my road to happiness.

I would like to have children and teach them how to live in an effective way so they might understand my words and follow my <u>example</u> and words.

I want to gain a perfect knowledge of the gospel, gaining a testimony in every important aspect of the gospel.

Always be thin.

<u>Write about your determination to do what you believe.</u>

Mar. 23, 1993. Today I cried hard for the first time and felt so bad for feeling the way I did. Why can't I just do what's right--pray, read scriptures, exercise and stop wallowing in my own weaknesses and sins. It's almost as though I must enjoy the pain.

I tell myself that I can't find the strength to do as I

should. I have to find the power within myself to start to change. Brian cannot do it for me. He can't force me to and he can't know exactly what I need. God is the only one that does and somewhere inside myself I do, too.

Reflect on how you are doing. Write any new insights, growth gained, how you're overcoming. List any changes needed to achieve your goals. Describe increased gratitude and determination to continue.

Sept. 13, 1984. It's hard to believe I'm writing in a new journal once more. Time goes by so fast and I feel overwhelmed by the fact that days pass me by and I can hardly see a change in my self until I look and read in my journal. Then I see I'm growing spiritually and I know I'm progressing.

Read your journal aloud in therapy, to a friend, even to yourself. This will strengthen the feeling of your words.

After you use your journal to help you heal, you will see a difference in the way you look at your past. As you examine your pain, you will find the experience still exists but it is completely changed.

Cautions about expressing pain in your journal.
It may not be best to leave some writing for others such as graphic abuse experiences or deep confusing emotions you sort through. Allow yourself to write about these experiences as you work through the issues. Then permit yourself and your inner child to do with them what would help you heal such as burn or shred them, send them away in a helium balloon, or mail them to a perpetrator.

Some writing is only to release pain so you can be

eased of the pain trapped inside. To remember it forever in a journal may only keep you holding onto deep pain from which the Savior longs for you to be freed by giving the burden to Him.

The legacy of a journal. Maybe you are lucky enough to possess an ancestor's journal. Many of our ancestors suffered painful experiences. Because they kept a diary, we have their experiences today. Years later, we can benefit from their experiences. When you write about your experiences, your pain, your progress and your setbacks, you leave a legacy for others.

As you use your journal to heal, you leave another tangible legacy--a healed mother, sister, daughter, wife. This enables you to help build a life for the next generation free from abuse and unhealthy traditions.

Journal writing is beneficial to healing. You will come to understand your feelings better as you write because they will be clarified as you ponder and analyze. Journal writing will help you examine your life as it is and set goals for how you hope it will be in the future.

Conclusion
1. Journals are a way to analyze life clearly and honestly, to set goals to change behavior.
2. You can change your feelings about experiences as you analyze them in your journal.
3. You leave a written legacy when you write in a journal.

CHAPTER SEVEN

PURE GOLD LIKE UNTO CLEAR GLASS

"And God shall wipe away all tears from their eyes; and there shall be no more death, neither sorrow, nor crying, neither shall there be any more pain. . .

"He that overcometh shall inherit all things. . . that great city. . . And the city was pure gold, like unto clear glass" (Rev. 21:4, 7, 10, 18).

As we present our pain to the Savior He will comfort, heal us, and give us the greatest gift of heaven--peace. God will melt us from shattered glass to make us whole, so now will He give us heaven's purified gold. Just as gold is purified in the refiner's fire and made into its most precious form, so is broken glass melted and made into its perfect state to clearly reflect truth in its purity and light.

We are as a city. Each inner part is who we are. Once each part is taught truth to become whole, all parts become one great whole making an organized functioning entity. We are complex, yet simple in purity and beauty, as God's hand refines and guides our understanding and heart to His loving ways.

God's glory shines through us as His Atonement burns through our souls revealing our precious worth as His own. As we overcome all with Him, He gives us His endless mercy as inheritance. The Atonement of our Savior heals our broken hearts and we show our gratitude to Him as we come to Him and accept His love and sacrifice. We give glory and honor to Him who made us whole.

GRATITUDE

What does gratitude have to do with healing?
My life feels rotten, how can I feel gratitude?

Gratitude adds a magical power to healing. It is a way of allowing yourself to have an outlook of hope. It is a way of looking at good as you turn your eyes away from pain for a moment.

Feeling gratitude about your childhood is healing. Look back at each good event from your childhood. Do you remember times of despair followed by times you felt an easing of your pain? Think of a good friend who came into your life. Recall a prayer that was answered or a time you were given a feeling of peace.

You may feel that there was nothing good in your childhood, but this is never the case. There is opposition in all things. We all experience bad, but we also experience good.

Even if you don't feel gratitude, you can desire it. Act as if you feel gratitude and eventually you will feel it. Healing moves more quickly when you are grateful.

Gratitude can ease your pain. I remember calling to God as I prayed in my heart, "I feel so much pain. Help me. What should I do? I need someone to help me." This seemed to intensify the anxiety I was feeling. I was focusing on the pain. It was intense and I made it worse by screaming to God to fulfill my needs. I asked, "Why won't God help me? Does He think I deserve this? I must deserve this."

Then a thought came, *What has God done for you already?* I searched to remember, then answered, "Thank you for when you answered my prayer. Thank you for the peaceful times. Thank you for this person in my life who is a strength to me. Thank you for my therapist who tries to help me. I am grateful to have resources to help me sort out this insanity. I'm grateful I can keep functioning. I'm grateful this is not really happening all over again. I'm grateful I'm free to choose for myself now."

I expressed gratitude for anything for which I was grateful. God eased my pain and increased my gratitude. Gratitude gave my pain something else on which to focus. Gratitude blessed me to work with my anxiety and not fight it. It was like magic in that it increased my ability to move forward to heal.

Feel gratitude for life itself. I learned another lesson about gratitude when our six-month-old daughter, BreAnne, had her first of three surgeries. Her sister, Katilyn, became ill the night before my husband and I were to take BreAnne to the hospital.

After a long night, I woke realizing I had to take BreAnne to the hospital alone while my husband stayed home and cared for Katilyn. My heart sank. I knew I couldn't get through the twelve hour preparation of I.V.'s, tubes, and blood work, then the 3 hour surgery and five day stay without the Lord's help. I prayed, "I'm alone. I can't do this without you. Please stay with me."

At the hospital BreAnn started with stomach pumping and blood work. Then came the time for the I.V.'s. The nurses couldn't get them to work though they tried again and again. I sat by my crying baby saying, "I'm sorry this is such a bad day. This is no fun. I'm so sorry."

Finally, they made me leave. As I walked down the hall with tears in my eyes, hearing my baby scream in pain from that little room, a thought came to me, *This life is so full of incredible pain--so full of hard experiences, yet I would not want to change it for anything in the world. I have learned so much about God. He sees all our pain for a purpose. Even at its worst, life is beautiful. I am grateful just to experience life. I am grateful to be a part of all of this.* I felt a sweet peace from feeling gratitude in the midst of pain.

There is power in gratitude. Jesus taught the healing power of gratitude. He healed ten lepers and sent them to the priests.

"And one of them, when he saw that he was healed, turned back, and with a loud voice glorified God,

"And fell down on his face at his feet, giving him thanks: and he was a Samaritan.

"And Jesus answering said, Were there not ten cleansed? but where are the nine?

"There are not found that returned to give glory to God, save this stranger.

"And he said unto him, Arise, go thy way: thy faith hath made thee whole" (Luke 17:15-19).

It takes faith to show gratitude, faith to believe that God really does care, that the good you see comes from Him. This scripture shows that not only did the leper receive physical healing in the beginning with the other nine, but he received a spiritual wholeness from God that comes from recognizing God's hand in the healing process. Being whole means being complete. I believe as we heal emotionally, we can also heal spiritually and become whole through gratitude for our Savior.

What can you do to feel and show gratitude?
- Express gratitude in your prayers.
- Keep a journal to help you see God's hand in your life.
- Write in your journal about God's goodness to you.
- Write a note to someone who has had an impact on your life.

- Share with someone the events in your life for which you feel grateful.

When you are in the midst of pain, it is difficult to think about being grateful. But as you look for the blessings in your life, you will discover more blessings. Your healing will progress more quickly and you will find joy in life as you heal.

Conclusion:

1. Even in bad times, it is healing to look for good in your life.

2. You can be grateful for life itself.

3. Gratitude helps heal the body and spirit.

PRAYING WITH GRATITUDE AND REAL INTENT

Is there anything I can do to make prayer easier?

How do I really pray and not simply go through the motions?

Prayer can be such a difficult process that it is a relief to find anything to make it easier. Maybe you can relax a little when you realize that the most important aspect of prayer is not the formality of it. God cares that you are praying sincerely from your heart.

It was natural for me to pray in my heart continually, because every minute was difficult. Prayer was like talking to a a friend at my side, someone who cared and shared my life with me.

My prayers were like a conversation, "Help me discover what I need to do. Help me open my mind to think clearly. Help me think clearly enough to find something at the store. Help me so I don't feel I'm making a fool out myself. Help me relax. Please bless me to recognize how to get through this day. Thank you, Father."

I learned how to pray continually for myself and others, and to show gratitude for prayers answered. I know God heard and answered those heartfelt prayers. Prayer helped me mend my broken heart. To me, the most vital part of healing was discovering the power of my prayers.

Pray with real intent. Like Moses, when he parted the Red Sea, you have to seek with real intent. You need a sense of urgency. The Israelites would have been destroyed by Pharaoh's soldiers had they not prayed with urgency. With real intent, you can recognize and receive revelation so you can survive spiritually.

If your prayers are casual, your eyes may be closed to see God's direction. You may not hear His counsel. God may not give answers or may choose to be slow to answer when you act like you don't care or pretend it doesn't really matter. When you seek with a sincere heart, you can recognize answers to your prayers.

"For I know the thoughts that I think toward you, saith the Lord, thoughts of peace, and not of evil, to give you an expected end.

"Then shall ye call upon me, and ye shall go and pray unto me, and I will hearken unto you.

"And ye shall seek me, and find me, when ye shall search for me with all your heart.

"And I will be found of you, saith the Lord: and I will turn away your captivity, and I will gather you from all the nations, . . .and I will bring you again into the place whence I caused you to be carried away captive" (Jeremiah 29:11-14).

Please pray. Pray with all your energy of heart. Don't simply go through the motions. God will answer your prayers and reveal the answers to "mysteries" you need to unlock.

Your prayers will unlock the mysteries of heaven for you! Through prayer you can learn the mysteries that will enable you to heal. You have assurance God will reveal things that have never before been revealed. You can tap into God's infinite wisdom.

Pray with gratitude. I discovered that revelation or blessings would continue if I thanked God for what He had done. I found that showing gratitude filled my heart with the Holy Ghost. I could again receive a witness that what I had experienced really was from God, that He loved me, and that He would continue to help me. Showing gratitude for God's direction and help would soften my heart towards God and keep the line of communication open between us.

Apr. 17, 1996. I'm getting closer to being in "the path, the way." I'm feeling more internally connected. It feels so peaceful and calming to pray. I went to therapy last Thursday and my therapist told me to thank God for every step of healing.

Praying with the attitude of gratitude has increased my closeness with God in ways I was yearning for. My desire to hunger and thirst after righteousness has helped me to rediscover the power of the scriptures as well.

If you just ask for help, work to receive help, then receive help, God is doing all the giving. Showing gratitude then feeling God's love binds you together. It is the blessing of prayer that breaks barriers, softens the heart, and brings true joy into your life.

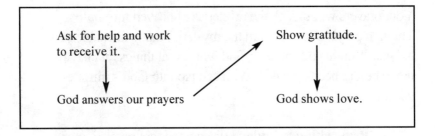

Prayer, though difficult, is essential to healing. Start where you are and attempt to communicate with God. Pray wherever and however you can.

Try to believe that a loving God wants to hear from you. Then express your gratitude to God for the difference you see in your life. As you do this you will feel deep gratitude and receive God's nurturing love.

Conclusion
1. You must pray with real intent to enlist God's help in your healing.
2. When you pray with gratitude and real intent, you bond with Heavenly Father and feel His love.

IRONIC SIMILARITIES BETWEEN REPENTING AND HEALING
Why do I feel pain and guilt when I didn't do anything wrong?
Do my feelings of guilt mean I need to repent?

The inner turmoil you feel from abuse may cause distorted thinking. Perhaps you feel or have felt responsibility for your perpetrator. Your shame and guilt may have caused a distorted view of who is responsible for what happened.

As an abuse victim, you may be confused about what

you should do to feel peace. If you feel guilt and shame about the abuse, you may feel you need to repent so the feelings of guilt and shame will go away. Many abuse victims are chronic "repenters." (See *Perfectionism, p. 27; Guilt, p. 220.*)

July 27, 1993. Tonight I feel so humbled. The last few days as I've sincerely studied the scriptures, my weaknesses have played repeatedly through my mind and heart. I keep thinking to myself, "Today I'll do better." Not only am I not doing better, but I'm doing worse. My weaknesses seem to manifest themselves to me in a magnified way.

Tonight I feel so sorry for my sins. I'm so sorry I think I can do better all by myself. I want to do better through the Savior. I am so sorry. I desire to be purified and sanctified through the Savior.

Repenting doesn't work, however. You cannot repent for someone else's sin. Thus, you are left with the same guilty feelings. You may begin to think that you will feel unworthy and unclean no matter what you do.

How repenting and healing are alike. Ironically, repentance and healing do have similarities:
- Sin, whether you commit the sin or the sin is committed upon you, both cause pain and inner turmoil.
- The Atonement of the Savior encompasses both. Both cases have the same end result--peace.

Repentance is necessary for the adult self to gain peace after committing a sin. However, to find peace after abuse, the inner child must heal. A person who sins and then repents is cleansed and freed from the "chains of hell" the actions created. The person must get on the path of righteous living. Time is lost.

A person who heals from abuse is freed from inner turmoil and the sinner's act. Now the victim can continue on the path back to Heavenly Father. With the healing process you have continual progression. You learn about Heavenly Father with every step. As you heal you are freed to internalize truth and act on that truth without the restrictions of inner pain.

Are your sins connected to your abuse? Your abuse may have weakened your ability to choose correctly as an adult. You may struggle with sexuality, honesty, or some other problem. You may want to make good choices but are limited in acting upon your desires. (See *Second Sins, p. 171; Sexual Boundaries, p. 180.*)

Stop mercilessly beating yourself up for the actions caused by the abuse. Take responsibility as an adult and go back to the core problem and take care of the broken child within. Your secondary problems will start to dissipate as your beliefs and feelings heal. (See *Strengthening against Damaging Cycles, p. 260.*)

As your adult self continues to repent of the present sins related to everyday living and your inner child continues to move forward to heal, the Savior's Atonement will engulf all of the pain you experience.

As adults we all commit sins and need to repent. Children, however, are innocent. As you recognize which part of yourself is responsible for your actions you can move toward the Savior's gift of peace through repentance and healing.

Conclusion:

1. Abuse victims desire to feel peace. This will not come from repenting for the perpetrator's actions. Peace comes from healing.

2. There are similarities between repentance and

healing. Both lead to peace, both lead to a release from the effects of sin.

3. Perpetrators can repent and start on the right path. Victims can heal and continue on the path. Every step is progression.

WHY GOD'S POWER IS GREATER THAN SATAN'S
Do I have hope if I suffered from Satanic abuse?
Is it possible to get out of Satan's grasp?

Satan wants you to believe he is more powerful than God. Satan is real and so is his power, but Heavenly Father is Omnipotent. God has all power. If you turn to God and remain on His side, you are with the greatest source of power. Lucifer shrinks before that power. If you become a friend to God and stay on His side, Satan has <u>no</u> power over you.

Satan's limitations. If you were to see Satan, you would be surprised at his insignificance or lack of <u>power</u>. You would ask in disbelief if he was the one who caused all the problems on earth.

"They that see thee shall narrowly look upon thee, and consider thee, saying, Is this the man that made the earth to tremble, that did shake kingdoms;

"That made the world as a wilderness, and destroyed the cities thereof; that opened not the house of his prisoners?" (Isa. 14:16-17).

Satan may seem powerful, but he has limitations. He works using power within strict limits allowed by the laws of agency. This is why he'll be bound someday.

Satan takes God's beautiful ways and twists the truth to create Satanic ways. He uses loud scare tactics. When people with the power of God stand up to Satan, he is subjected to and must shrink and disappear before deity.

Sept. 17, 1991. I went to a quiet spot to meditate and pray today. As I prayed, I realized I was in the center of a spot that was used for Satanic worship. I received a witness that God's power overrides Satan's so that only God's influence will be felt if you are seeking Him. I felt the Holy Ghost present and no influence of the adversary.

When I was struggling to understand God's power versus Satan's power, I thought of the movie "The Wizard of Oz." Dorothy and her friends were shaking before the great wizard when Dorothy's little dog revealed a man behind a curtain. He was not the powerful man the travelers supposed him to be. He was limited to do only what Dorothy and her friends believed he could do. Satan is like the wizard.

Eternally, Satan has only the power over you that you give him through your agency. He has power when you decide to follow, be fearful, or be controlled by his devices. The more energy you use to be close to God, the less power Satan has. The Savior was tempted by Satan. He suffered temptations but did not heed them. You can follow the Savior's example and Satan will have no influence over you.

Look to the Savior to overcome Satan. In *"Willingness to Heal"* (p. 58) you can read how poisonous serpents bit the Israelites, then Moses raised a brazen serpent which represented the Savior who would heal them.

Moses was commanded to hold up the rod because he was a prophet, a witness of Christ. The poisonous snakes represented Satan. Symbolically, the Israelites were poisoned by Satan. To heal, the Israelites were to lift their eyes to the rod. They did this if they had faith it would heal them.

You too must do your part having faith that the Savior will heal you. He will. I promise. I know.

Satan inflicted our Savior with all the pain hell had to offer. You may see flashes of horror you experienced and feel you are engulfed in Satan's wicked poison. The Savior overcame all the poison from the snake and has risen above all evil. He has been lifted up. That is why you and I don't need to fear Satan.

Satan may cause you pain. His poison may feel intensely overwhelming to you, but if you look to the Savior who overcame and conquered Satan's power, then you too can overcome pain as the Savior did.

The Savior's Atonement encompasses all pain and suffering because He suffered for all of it. Satan is nothing to fear, but the Savior has everything to embrace. I know this is true.

I love the Savior with all my heart. I know He makes broken souls whole. He has no boundaries on what He can heal. He was bruised, broken, and torn for you. You too may know how it feels to be bruised, broken, and torn. But you can be assured that Christ understands your pain. He has experienced <u>all</u> hell had to offer because of His love for you. He overcame it all.

Before Christ engulfs your pain in peace, you experience a taste of the pain that He went through. This way you come to know the Savior and become a little like Him. What a miraculous gift, what an indescribable honor. What a beautiful, merciful God. Isn't this why we are here on earth? We gain experience and try to become like the Savior, so we can return to the Father.

"Then shall the dust return to the earth as it was: and the spirit shall return unto God who gave it" (Eccl. 12:7).

291

Satanic Influences. You can overcome the influence of Satan's power, Satanic ways, evil practices and traditions. If you experienced Satanic abuse, this does not make you evil. (See *Shame, p. 224.*)

Realize you chose Heavenly Father's side before you came to earth (see Rev. 12:7-9). As you heal, recognizing that evil happened, this will only enable you to experience the opposite and love the Savior more.

As far as I can distinguish, everything that Satan uses to pull people down to hell was first created by God. God governs all truth and Satan takes God's truth and subtly twists it into lies. This twisting of truths and power is the only power Satan is enabled. Satan twists everything good by making subtle changes until it is completely wrong.

This discovery helped me to realize who is all powerful. Satan has limitations to his power. His greatest limitation comes when we reject his ways and cling to God's ways.

We learn of Satan's limitation of power in the scriptures. "And Moses and Aaron went in unto Pharoah . . . .and Aaron cast down his rod before Pharaoh, and before his servants, and it became a serpent" (Ex. 7:10).

Pharoah used the adversary's power which were wise men and sorcerers. "For they cast down every man his rod, and they became serpents: but Aaron's rod swallowed up their rods" (v. 12). God's power was stronger than Satan's.

You don't need to fear Satan. He will be overcome when you cast out fear through faith in the Savior, Jesus Christ and cling to truth. I promise you that if you will do this, you will never be overpowered by the evil one.

Conclusion:

1. God is more powerful than Satan.

2. Christ overcame Satan's power.

3. Your suffering will lead you to be more like the Savior.

UNDERSTANDING SUFFERING

Why must I suffer if the Savior already suffered for my pain?

If I do suffer, does that mean I have not accepted the Savior's Atonement?

Suffering can be a difficult concept to understand. Many people have the mistaken idea that if they suffer, it is a punishment from God. Others may think if they feel pain and sorrow it means they don't believe in the Atonement and Christ's suffering for us. Still others may think it is best to bury sorrow and get on with life. What do you believe?

Myths about suffering. Here are a few misconceptions about how to view pain and suffering.

1. Myth: Weak people cry. Strong people don't let adversity affect them.

Truth: It takes courage and strength to allow yourself to be humble and submissive and feel pain.

2. Myth: I can't struggle. I have to be strong to help others.

Truth: If you do not suffer for yourself, you give your suffering to others. Others learn to go through their trials by your example.

3. Myth: If I allow myself to feel pain, it will be more than I can handle. It will engulf me and I may not be able to handle it.

Truth: If you do not suffer your own pain, you are left on your own trying to hold back, and control what is trying to surface. This takes a lot of energy. If you allow or embrace the pain, God will take anything beyond what you can endure. Your pain will turn to joy and peace because of the Atonement.

4. *Myth:* The Savior atoned for suffering, so I do not need to suffer. He already suffered for me.

Truth: If you did not accept sacrifice through suffering, you could not be a witness of tasting Christ's sacrifice and stand as God's servant (see 2 Cor. 1:5-6). You could not be a true follower and could not claim to take His name upon you. Your endurance brings salvation.

5. *Myth:* I've heard I should give my pain to the Savior. If I feel pain have I failed to give it to the Savior?

Truth: You cannot give to the Savior something you have not held in your own hands. You must hold some of your own suffering before you can give it to Him. Going through painful experiences does not mean you are not including the Savior. You protect yourself from pain until you are ready to handle it. You must learn as you face and endure some of your pain before the Savior takes the rest.

6. *Myth:* I've tried to do what God asked and I still feel pain. Does this mean I deserve to feel pain, that God does not love me, or I'm not worthy for His Atonement to help me?

Truth: God allows you to feel pain because without suffering, challenges, and trials your spirit would not grow in this life and you would not obtain higher levels of spiritual growth. Your spiritual capacity is strengthened when you continue to endure during prolonged pain. This is how you are formed to perfection:

"For thou art my servant: I have formed thee; thou art my servant: O Israel, thou shalt not be forgotten of me" (Isa.

44:21).

Even though your pain continues, there will be times when you find an easing which will allow the pain to be bearable. Like broken glass, some melting is required to weld the pieces to one again. God will not forget you as you endure in pain.

Why must you look to God when you are suffering?

- The Savior can help you to stretch beyond what you think you can.
- God will take your willingness and mold you to your greatest potential.
- You can learn personally who He is that suffered all.
- God will comfort you, then you can comfort others unconditionally without judgment.
- Through God you will know joy because you have experienced pain, the opposite of joy.

How can you know if you are accepting the Savior's Atonement?

- You don't quit because you believe the mercy of the Savior will encompass the pain you're experiencing.
- You seek and apply truths from pure sources--scriptures and the guidance of God through prayer. You recognize truths which are reiterated and defined in good books and counsel you are given.
- You learn to recognize and follow the direction of God's Holy Spirit to find people, conditions and experiences that will help you heal.
- As you face pain you show gratitude to God for what you have. You are cultivating a spirit of humility recognizing goodness from God.

By understanding the truth about suffering and how it guides you to healing, you can resist fighting pain. Strive to accept and apply principles of truth that will invite the Savior to assist you in your healing. God loves you. He wants you to find peace and joy. He will guide you as you welcome His influencing hand.

Conclusion:

1. If you allow yourself to suffer, you will be able to work through your pain.

2. God allows you to feel pain so you can grow. You have not rejected the Atonement because you feel pain and sorrow.

WHY WE EXPERIENCE SUFFERING, PAIN, AND SORROW

Why does God allow suffering to happen?
What is the purpose of suffering?

No one wants to suffer or feel pain. We hope for a life of joy and happiness that is free from sorrow. It is not easy for God to see us suffer but He allows it to happen for several reasons. We came to earth to learn as we experience opposition. We suffer so we can grow and learn and become like Job, "perfect and upright" (Job 1:1).

Internal pain purifies and sanctifies. Sometimes it is only through pain and suffering that we get to know God. The result of suffering can be good. Suffering can sanctify and purify. For Jonah, affliction came to purify and sanctify him in preparing him to serve God.

Jonah said, "I cried by reason of my affliction unto the Lord, and he heard me; out of the belly of hell cried I, and thou heardest my voice.

"When my soul fainted within me I remembered the Lord: and my prayer came in unto thee . . . I will sacrifice unto thee with the voice of thanksgiving; I will pay that that I have vowed" (Jonah 2:2,7,9).

A personal example. I had an experience that taught me many things about why we suffer. One day I could not function and felt an intense feeling of despair. I tried to find a peaceful setting to ease my anxiety and hopeless feelings. I lay on a blanket in the sunshine to absorb goodness and warmth. None came.

My anxiety and despair intensified and I felt as though I would be swallowed up in impenetrable suffering. It was as though all of the sorrow caused by those who had abused me throughout my life was culminating into one great whole within me. I searched for how to be released, how to escape, or how to work through the pain. No answer seemed to come. I had no resources on my own to be lifted out of the pain.

I started to desperately fight the pain. I panicked thinking maybe I would never escape the indescribable hole. I believed dying would be my only way out.

My husband came to my side trying to soothe my pain. His touch only intensified it and seemed to deepen my darkness. Maybe dying was the answer to the dilemma and my only escape.

In a peaceful voice I heard Brian ask me to relax and I focused on that. Then a thought came, *Where is this Jesus who has suffered for my suffering? Where is the Savior who has saved us from the pain of the world? Where is He that He might bind my spirit's sorrow?*

I asked Brian to pray for me. He carried me in the house and held me as he prayed for me. He said he felt I could endure this and God expected me to endure it. As I did, my pain would ease.

I accepted the pain and allowed it to be there. As I did, I was freed a little. Then I had more energy to deal with it. I began to see a light within myself that came and slowly eased the intensity of my grief. Then I felt the pain slowly drain out of me.

I fell asleep for a short time, then was able to get up and function. I was prompted to call a friend and help her with a problem. It was awe provoking to me that I could help her so shortly after going through tremendous pain of my own. Experiencing my pain actually blessed me to help someone else.

Suffering and agency. I learned several important principles from this experience. Most fundamental is this: Suffering is part of this world because of the opposition caused from the use of agency. All men and women are endowed with agency when they come into this life. Agency is a most precious gift.

Even the Savior chose to endure suffering using His agency to do as His Father willed. "O my Father, if it be possible, let this cup pass from me: nevertheless not as I will, but as thou wilt" (Matt. 26:39).

People make wrong choices because they have agency. These choices cause pain and suffering--not only for themselves, but for others as well. We do not suffer because God has turned His back on us. We suffer because someone has used agency unwisely.

Suffering as the Savior suffered. The Savior did not experience pain as a punishment for doing wrong. He chose to suffer because He loved us so much. "For Christ is the end of the law for righteousness to every one that believeth" (Rom.

10:4).

When you are innocent and suffer pain because of another's acts, you are experiencing a degree of what the Savior suffered. (See *The Savior's Suffering, Pain, and Sorrow [The Atonement], p. 306.*)

Enduring pain and sorrow. God knows what you are made of. He knows you have what it takes to heal and endure. You learn this for yourself as you suffer. You learn (and gain) your strengths in your endurance. This might be one of the reasons James wrote, "Behold, we count them happy which endure" (James 5:11).

God promises you won't be given more than you can endure, but this doesn't mean that sometimes you won't need to be strengthened. The Savior himself needed strengthening as He suffered in the Garden of Gethsemane. "And there appeared an angel unto him from heaven, strengthening him" (Luke 22:43). God sent an angel to minister to Him.

Imagine unseen angels there strengthening you. I believe they are there. I have seen and felt them for myself and others.

You learn as you suffer that if you fight physical pain, it gets worse. When I didn't fight mental turmoil, I could handle it better. When I accepted the pain and allowed it to be a part of me, I had more energy to deal with the pain and it slowly eased.

July 17, 1994. A couple of weeks ago Brian said to turn to the Savior's Atonement. I felt baffled by the thought.

I know the Savior (because of the Atonement) carries my burden when it is more than I can stand. I want my suffering to be for my growth so I am going to seek help to be able to bear the burden better rather than simply get relief. I need a therapist soon so I can see more clearly what I can do to heal.

Learning to know God through suffering. When you face pain and accept the challenge to hold it, work through it, and let its effects go through you, you taste what the Savior went through. This gives you a feeling of amazement about the Lord's love. Your love for Him will become undying and your understanding of who you are will bring you to God. You will feel a kinship, a friendship, a loyalty to God. (See *Suffering Is a Catalyst to Eternal Growth, p. 304.*)

Oct. 1, 1995. I've been through a lot spiritually since I started this journal. The Savior has shown me a great deal of His healing power. I feel as though the pain, confusion and fear have been eased, if not dissolved.

My faith in the Savior has increased, thus fear has subsided. Confusion has been replaced with understanding (not necessarily logical, but spiritual), and pain has been validated, felt, eased and healed.

The Savior is more real to me. I love Him. My scripture study and prayer are more consistent and sincere and I feel the Holy Ghost's peace and guidance more often. The process of change has been slow but very significant and I love God so much for helping me. I feel I am becoming stronger. I am so grateful.

Suffering gives us experience. To Jeremiah the word of the Lord came saying, "Before I formed thee in the belly I knew thee" (Jeremiah 1:5). We all knew God and He knew us before our birth. God knew what we were made of and what we could endure in this life. I believe we all wanted to gain the experience of earth life, but we are often shocked at what we must endure.

Eliphaz counseled Job stating, "Yet man is born unto trouble, as the sparks fly upward.

"I would seek unto God, and unto God would I commit my cause" (Job 5:7-8).

We forget that gaining experience is a necessary key to what moves us toward heaven. God will give us choices and experiences to see if we will do whatever He commands. God knows that all things give us experience and are for our good.

Our Father in Heaven believes in experience. He knows we must be tested and tried so we can become perfect like God. "Be ye therefore perfect, even as your father which is in heaven is perfect" (Matt. 5:48). As we suffer, we choose who we really will be and of what stuff we will be made.

July 2, 1995. Today as we sat in church Brian told me I looked beautiful. Then he asked, "Do you know what it is that makes you so beautiful? It's not having so much pain weighing you down from your abuse issues."

My mind and eyes flowing, I thought of how long and hard I had worked through pain and how many times I'd felt it would never end. How crazy I felt at times, how alone and confused, and how going back to one more therapist seemed more than I wanted to do. But with Brian's support, prayers, and belief in me I went back again to see if I could face and let go of the pain.

How grateful I am to God. Things did not come in my time--not in any way. But He has blessed me line upon line and like never before I understand a lot better what inner calmness, love, and forgiveness are. I saw in my mind's eye, the Savior redeeming my soul as a child and now He redeems me from the pain. How I love God!

Heavenly Father has taught me of His mercy and eternal love. I know God loves me unconditionally and knowing this gives me hope to overcome and to go forward toward Him.

For so long I have struggled to see things clearly. My past pain has filled my life with distorted beliefs and theories and many times my experiences showed my beliefs to be valid. I am learning to see things through new eyes. I believe that this is not a talent or a skill I'm working on. I truly believe it is a gift or blessing of healing from God.

Through suffering you gain empathy for others. Our Father in Heaven and his Son teach you how to comfort others through the way they comfort you in your sorrow. Paul, who knew much about suffering, wrote:

"Blessed be God, even the Father of our Lord Jesus Christ, the Father of mercies, and the God of all comfort;

"Who comforteth us in all our tribulation, that we may be able to comfort them which are in any trouble, by the comfort wherewith we ourselves are comforted of God" (2 Cor. 1:3-4).

As you heal, you can care for others. You can listen to another's sorrow and feel empathy. You will be able to strengthen and help carry their burden because you have experienced burdens yourself.

Rewards come after the pain. You can feel comforted when you realize the goal in life is not to get <u>out</u> of the pain but to work through it. The Savior can teach you how to grow through your pain. You don't want to escape the pain and miss out on the growth and molding it will give you.

Pain is not only for the wicked, the wicked run from it. Pain is part of life. When you follow God you can turn to your pain to allow for it to mold you as clay as God would have you. When you look back on life, your most treasured moments will be when you, with the help of God, triumphed over those trials that seemed impossible to overcome.

John the Revelator saw hosts of exalted beings and described them this way, "There are they which came out of great tribulation, and have washed their robes, and made them white in the blood of the Lamb.

"Therefore are they before the throne of God, and serve him day and night in his temple: and he that sitteth on the throne shall dwell among them.

"They shall hunger no more, neither thirst any more; neither shall the sun light on them, nor any heat.

"For the Lamb which is in the midst of the throne shall feel them, and shall lead them unto living fountains of waters: and God shall wipe away all tears from their eyes" (Rev. 7:14-17).

When you come to the Savior to allow Him to heal you, you will discover that sorrow is a temporary condition. You can be healed through the Atonement. In time you will find yourself in a condition of inexpressible happiness as you live with your Father in Heaven in an exalted state.

Conclusion:

1. You are allowed to suffer so you can be like the Savior.

2. Much of the suffering in the world comes because God's children are allowed agency.

3. You will learn empathy through your suffering.

SUFFERING IS A CATALYST TO ETERNAL GROWTH

Doesn't suffering hold me back from progressing?
Why do I feel like a failure when I am in pain?

When you study the lives of God-fearing people in the scriptures and in our day, you can see a pattern in how they deal with pain and adversity. You can observe that as they stand on the edge of failure during periods of intense suffering, they are blessed with growth and success if they willingly endure their pain. As grief, pain and suffering are overcome, unspeakable joy is the reward.

Good people suffer and experience opposition.
Pain and adversity do not signify wickedness. Adam and Eve suffered the murder of their son, Abel. Abraham was a victim of his father's wickedness. Paul was imprisoned time after time. During suffering these valiant people fought an internal battle and endured long enough to triumph.

Suffering is not merely for correction. It is often a means to stretch your spirit to learn beyond what you could while being comfortable. Suffering is a catalyst which molds your spirit to learn to become like God. You learn to adjust your will to match God's when you suffer willingly and seek Him.

Suffering actually can cause you to rise to a higher level of righteousness, walking a step closer to your potential. Suffering helps you to become a little more like the Savior if you allow it to mold you, teach you, and guide you toward Him.

Growth through suffering. The following are some ways you will grow as you try to stay close to the Lord through your suffering:

304

<u>Repentance.</u> Through repentance you experience a cleansing process that enables growth. David sorrowed, "For I will declare mine iniquity; I will be sorry for my sin" (Ps. 38:18).

As adults we all sin and need daily repentance. Christ lamented over Jerusalem, "O Jerusalem, Jerusalem, . . . how often would I have gathered thy children together, even as a hen gathereth her chickens under her wings, and ye would not" (Matt. 23:37). When you repent you allow Christ to gather you. (See *What Ensures You as a Child Did Not Sin? p. 228; The Savior's Suffering Pain and Sorrow [The Atonement], p. 306*.)

<u>You become an instrument in God's hands.</u> Through your suffering, you can help others through their suffering. When you have suffered, you are blessed with increased empathy for others. (See *Helping Others, p. 72*.)

<u>Suffering helps teach obedience.</u> The Savior learned obedience through suffering. "Though he were a Son, yet learned he obedience by the things which he suffered" (Heb. 5:8). A loving, Holy Father will teach and train you through your afflictions.

<u>Having suffered, you come to know Christ and the Father.</u> As you feel the pain of opposition in this life, you can learn to become one with God the Father and the Son (see John 17:11).

<u>You can gain the joys of heaven.</u> You become joint-heirs or one with Christ, worthy to be spiritually begotten. "And if children, then heirs; heirs of God, and joint-heirs with Christ; if so be that we suffer him, that we may be also glorified together" (Rom. 8:17).

You will grow line upon line as you learn to accept suffering patiently and submissively, trusting that God knows all and will consecrate your performance for your good. Suffering will allow you to overcome the "natural man" and will enable you to feel gratitude to God for His mercy through the Savior.

When I look back at my life, I have found the times I suffered the most while striving to be near God have been cherished moments of triumph. The amazing irony is that it was when I felt I was at my weakest moment, I was truly at my greatest.

God will open your eyes to spiritual understanding and strengthen you to walk with more precision toward Him on His path. More than anything, because of experiencing some of what He has experienced, you will be worthy to be called His and to be more like Him.

Conclusion:

1. Rain falls on the just and the unjust. In other words, righteous and wicked people experience suffering.

2. You can grow and become like the Savior if you suffer willingly.

3. The Savior will help you endure your suffering.

THE SAVIOR'S SUFFERING, PAIN, AND SORROW (The Atonement)

How can the Atonement help me?

What do I need to do to make the Atonement effective for me?

The Savior's Atonement was the greatest event in the history of the world. Through Christ's sacrifice the sins of the world were paid. Christ suffered for your sins, your pain, and your sorrow. He understands your pain perfectly because He suffered the magnitude of each and every sin and sorrow you will ever experience.

306

The Savior has suffered for your sins, pains, and sorrows. In a miraculous way our Savior paid for all sins and suffered for all pains and sorrows. He took upon Himself the pains of death so that we might be freed from the bands of death.

"Wherefore in all things it behoved him to be made like unto his brethren, that he might be a merciful and faithful high priest in things pertaining to God, to make reconciliation for the sins of the people.

"For in that he himself hath suffered being tempted, he is able to succour them that are tempted" (Heb.2:18).

We do not completely understand what happened in the Garden of Gethsemane, but Christ's suffering is described, "And being in an agony he prayed more earnestly: and his sweat was as it were great drops of blood falling down to the ground" (Luke 22:44).

The Savior alone can succor you in your suffering. When you are in pain, you can be assured that the Savior will understand your needs.

How do you make the Atonement operative in your life? In the New Testament Jesus gives a pattern on how to be healed: He promises that when we are converted, he will heal our broken hearts (see Matt. 13:15). He mourns that the people will not be converted so He can heal them.

Jesus calls all people to repent. All accountable adults have sinned and the Lord cannot look upon sin with the least degree of allowance. We all must daily evaluate, recommitting ourselves to repent and be converted because only the Savior is without sin. This is the pattern for the Savior's Atonement to heal us.

"He hath shewed thee, O man, what is good; and what doth the Lord require of thee, but to do justly, and to love mercy, and to walk humbly with thy God?" (Micah 6:8).

The Savior's arm of mercy is extended as an open invitation to come to Him. He won't pull us unwillingly from where we are. We must ask, seek, and knock. We must first do our part to find Him and then He will be there to walk with us.

May 24, 1990. I am so grateful to my Heavenly Father. I know He loves me. I know that He knows where I am and He is blessing my efforts to become a better person. I am grateful for my trials. They help me to stretch spiritually to become closer to God and to be humble and submissive. They also help me to become more pure in heart and cleansed of my spiritual impurities.

I know I can get through and overcome the pain and damage that my childhood sexual abuse has caused. I can overcome this and get married and have a family someday. I'm not sure how long it will take, but I know it can't take an eternity.

When the Savior suffered in the garden of Gethsemane, He suffered for this too. Somehow I must learn to give Him my pain so I may be free from it and that it may be swallowed up in His mercy and love. I am so grateful for the gospel of Jesus Christ. Where would I be without it? I love God. I will pray to always be near Him that I may feel of His love.

A broken heart and a contrite spirit. The Savior asks for a sacrifice, "The sacrifices of God are a broken spirit: a broken and a contrite heart" (Ps. 51:17). How can you offer a broken heart to the Savior? You can take your broken inner child to heal so she can feel peace and learn to love and trust her Savior. You can teach her truth helping her to be converted and gain a testimony of the Savior. (See *How Does God Ask Your Adult Self to View Your Inner Child? p. 217.*)

Your adult self must offer a sacrifice of a broken heart and a contrite spirit by striving to overcome through self mastery. This is how you make the Atonement effective in your life. You accept the Savior's complete mercy to your inner child for he said, "Suffer little children, and forbid them not, to come unto me: for of such is the kingdom of heaven" (Matt. 19:14).

As you love your inner child, guiding her to the Savior, you gain childlike attributes needed to enter the kingdom of God. Your adult self humbles herself to have a broken heart and a contrite spirit.

Why did the Savior come into the world? He came to save the world from all sin. He came into the world to save you from another person's sinful actions. You must put yourself in a position to accept His gift by being willing to work at healing and learning truth.

Come unto Christ as a little child. Your pain is real and the Savior offers a path to healing. You must literally come to Him as a little child. Your inner child seeks to know a Savior. Teach her about Jesus as you come to Him. You will be able to feel the full effect of the Atonement. (See *What Ensures You as a Child Did Not Sin? p. 228.*)

As you teach your inner child about the Savior you will become aware of her childlike attributes. Adults must always repent because we always fall short. As we do this and try to become as our beautiful inner child--innocent, pure, teachable-- we will attune ourselves to those things needed to inherit the kingdom of God.

I used to think because as a child I had experienced abuse, I as an adult could sit back and use my life's pain as an excuse for why I didn't seek Christ. I thought God would say on judgment day, "Julie Anne had an extremely hard package, I will give her a free ticket into heaven."

The price we pay to solicit the Atonement. The Savior's Atonement comes without money, but there is a price to pay. "Ho, every one that thirsteth, come ye to the waters, and he that hath no money; come ye, buy, and eat; yea, come, buy wine and milk without money and without price.

"Wherefore do ye spend money for that which is not bread? and your labour for that which satisfieth not? hearken diligently unto me, and eat ye that which is good, and let your soul delight itself in fatness" (Isa. 55:1-2).

You do not have to pay money. The Atonement is free to all, but if you want to be healed, you need to give your broken hearted inner child by hearkening--listening and obeying the words of God. You must also feast or internalize His way of living by allowing all that the Savior says and does to become a part of who you are.

Your suffering is a small portion of what Christ went through. It's an honor to go through pain like the Savior. The Savior didn't go through pain as a punishment for doing wrong. He innocently suffered showing great love for you. Christ offered Himself as a sacrifice for sin to answer the ends of the law to all those who have a broken heart and a contrite spirit. No one can take this from you. (See *Why We Experience Suffering, Pain, and Sorrow, p. 296*.)

When you look to the Savior, follow Him, and do all you can do, Christ's Atonement will envelop the rest. You must internally go to Him to be healed. The amazing thing about the Atonement is that all the words in the world cannot express the meaning the Atonement. The magnificent Savior of the world shares His word and His sacrifice with us.

Conclusion:

1. The Savior's Atonement is the pivotal event in the history of the world. In a way we do not understand, the Savior took upon Himself the pains and sins of all mankind.

2. The Savior has perfect empathy because He suffered for every sin, pain, and sorrow.

3. When you go to the Savior with a broken heart and a contrite spirit, He promises He will heal you.

AFTER THE STORM COMES THE RAINBOW

Some storms seem as though they will never end. I think Noah and his family felt the rain would never cease, the darkness would never break, and the flooded land would never dry. As I embarked on the beginning of my healing, I too could see nothing but storm and darkness. I felt I would be washed away with the flood of my new reality of pain and confusion.

I lived believing that somewhere I would find dry earth, sunlight and clear skies. Slowly it came. My painful storm erupted and calmed, then ceased.

I never realized what would follow. I only hoped for life to be as it used to be--life as I had known it. Now at the end of my healing I have found my rainbow. I have found what peace and joy can truly be like.

I never knew I could live life experiencing daily trials while within my heart I would feel a rainbow of continual joy and peace. Never again would I feel the pain of an inner child calling for refuge. My Savior has embraced my painful past and engulfed me in His Atoning love with the promise that never again shall my child self be molested or made afraid.

Never again will my spirit be darkened with the past evil acts of others. My inner children have been healed through the

Atonement of our great Redeemer. I am now free to feel and enjoy the blessing of the gospel promised to those who earnestly seek Him.

There are some gifts no person on earth can give us. Friends and loved ones may share wisdom, experience and great learning, but no one can heal our heart but God. Through the Holy Ghost God taught me who the Savior was. Then I was able to turn my pain over to Him.

The grossest mud was taken by my sweet friend and He gave me gold in return. I share some of that gold with you with the promise that you too may experience what I have. Jesus loves you and because He loves you, I can share all of this with you. Live as though there is a calm after the storm and you will find a rainbow.